From Zero to Zen

Zen /zen/

Adjective: peaceful and calm*

* It is my sincere hope this book brings you some peace of mind.

Praise for *From Zero to Zen*

"Reading *From Zero to Zen* is like sitting down with a friend who's been through the good, bad, and the ugly of caregiving and getting the inside scoop on everything you *really* need to know."

Jen Singer, author of *The Just Diagnosed Guides*

"As more of us deal with the reality of caring for aging parents, at a time when we are caring for our children, and our own mental health, Alexandra Free shows us a path toward calling in the best version of ourselves so we can cherish the last moments we have with our loved ones. Packed with you-don't-usually-know-it-until-it's-too-late information and compassionate support, *From Zero to Zen* is the friend we all need."

Ashleigh Renard, author of *Swing*

"Who doesn't need this book? If you are over 18 and live in the United States, buy a copy now. With absolute candor and clarity, Alexandra Free takes the reader through the aspects of caregiving no one ever talks about, including denial, grief, and paperwork. Checklists at the end of each chapter—and a free PDF on her website—leave you with plenty of next steps and a way to keep from feeling overwhelmed. This is the companion book that Atul Gawande's *Being Mortal* needed."

Stephanie Weaver, MPH, author of *The Migraine Relief Plan* and *The Migraine Relief Plan Cookbook*

"Think of *From Zero to Zen* as your roadmap to being a better caregiver for your loved one. The author, faced with both her dad's unexpected hospital stays and ten years of caring for her mother suffering from Alzheimer's, offers you not only practical knowledge but also the courage to embrace your journey. Ms. Free's candidness is refreshing, and the sharing of her story gives you the feeling you are not alone. If you are struggling with your journey as a caregiver, this book is packed with the guidance and caring you may be looking for at this very moment. This book is it."

Virginia Alice Crawford, author of *Honor One Another: The ABCs of Embracing Your Spirit Within*

"*From Zero to Zen* is the book that so many of us need right now. Filled with practical information and hard-won advice, this is the guide you'll want with you in the trenches of caregiving."

Aly Cohen, MD, author of *Non-Toxic: Guide to Living Healthy in a Chemical World*

"Anyone who might become a caregiver to a parent (which is to say, anyone) needs a copy of *From Zero to Zen*, Alexandra Free's invaluable guide to getting "all your ducks in a row" *before* there's a crisis. How many of us know our parents' blood type, for instance, or where the marriage license (or divorce agreement) is? How many of us even know *where* Mom or Dad stashed all the important documents, much less what counts as "important"?

As I read this book, I made a list of things to ask my own (still more-or-less) healthy parents and I'm grateful to Alexandra for this advice, all of which is clearly presented and grounded in her own experiences navigating the decline and death of her parents.

Reading this book is like having a conversation with your smartest, funniest friend, who reminds you not only to get that Durable Power of Attorney, but also that it's okay to feel frustrated or even angry with the difficulties of caregiving a parent. This wise friend also has generous and useful suggestions for the particular complexity of caring for parents with Alzheimer's.

Even if you think your parents have everything in order, you owe it to yourself to get this book—and maybe get a copy for your siblings, too. *From Zero to Zen* is an essential tool for navigating life as a caregiver with confidence and clarity."

Deborah Williams, Professor, Liberal Studies NYU, and author of *The Necessity of Young Adult Fiction*

A Guide to Help You Thrive as a Caregiver
(*from someone who's been there*)

From Zero to Zen

ALEXANDRA FREE

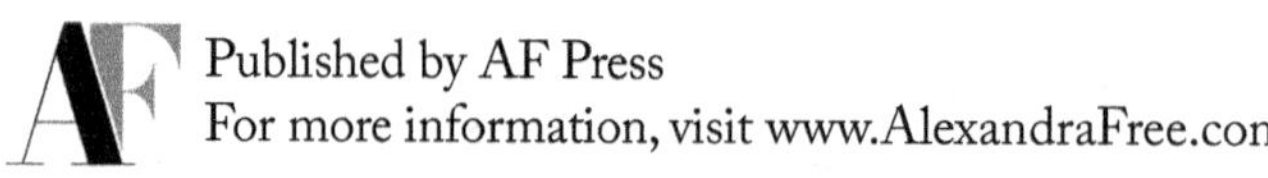

Published by AF Press
For more information, visit www.AlexandraFree.com

ISBN (paperback): 979-8-9884321-0-4
ISBN (ebook): 979-8-9884321-1-1

Book design by Christy Day, Constellation Book Services
Author photo by Kristen Driscoll

Printed in the United States of America

For Mom, Dad and Lola—I love and miss you.

And for all the caregivers out there
doing their best day in and day out—
I see you and you are amazing!

CONTENTS

Obstacles don't block the path,
they are the path.

– Zen proverb

I Went Through Hell
So You Don't Have To

Hello, friend. I'm glad you're here! Well, sort of. Let me explain…

The talented Toni Morrison once said, "If there's a book that you want to read, but it hasn't been written yet, then you must write it."

This is that book.

But this is also the book I wish I didn't have to write, and it's the book I truly hope you never need to read. However, it *is* the book I desperately could have used when I was caring for my sick parents, so I think that still falls within Ms. Morrison's purview.

You see, I believe none of us want our parents or loved ones to get sick, and we certainly don't lie awake at night excited by the prospect of becoming their caregivers. The fact is, people are living longer but unfortunately, they aren't living healthier—so the likelihood of becoming a caregiver to a sick and/or aging loved one is a very real possibility for all of us.

Until I started caring for my parents, I knew nothing—ZERO—about being a caregiver. I lived in Los Angeles, I had a career in television that I loved, and most everyone in my family lived until a ripe old age and died in their sleep. No one had debilitating illnesses, no one suffered, they were simply alive one minute and then dead the next.

While losing someone you love quickly is definitely heartbreaking and hard to process, I would ultimately learn what a gift it truly was. No one wants to stand by and watch someone they love suffer. Or, as is the case with a disease like Alzheimer's, watch as their loved one is robbed of the memories of the life they once had, slowly disappearing into the quicksand of nothingness.

I lost my beloved grandmother at the age of ninety-three. She spent the last day of her life chopping down a tree, hanging out with her pup, and being the healthy, independent badass I had always known her to be. She went to bed that night and basically, that was it. She was gone.

My father went next, a year later. But his story was very different. He entered the hospital for a minor surgery and seven painful, nightmarish months later, he finally passed away. As brutal as his story was, my mother's experience was worse.

My mother was diagnosed with Alzheimer's, and unlike my father who had a bevy of health issues, my mother remained healthy until the very end. Healthy, but rotting from the top down. As horrible as it was to watch my father slowly expire in a hospital bed, nothing compared to watching my brilliant, strong, independent mother disappear over a ten-year period, one brain cell at a time.

Prior to my parents' illnesses, I never thought about legal documents, I never worried about health insurance, I never had panic attacks about their finances. During my parents' illnesses, it felt like that was all I ever did.

I spent many days curled up in the fetal position in my bed, riddled with anxiety, praying for a miracle. On the days I wasn't doing that, I was talking with lawyers, accountants, elder care experts, and Medicaid counselors, learning everything I could to do what I needed to care for my parents and keep myself sane.

From Zero to Zen is the culmination of over a decade's worth of research coupled with my firsthand experience with the trials and tribulations of caregiving. It is my intention to share everything I've learned and experienced so that it can serve as a guide for how to go from being lost and overwhelmed to thriving as a caregiver. From documents you need, to information you must have, to self-care tips you should follow, it truly is the book I wish I had when I was where you are now.

The Chinese philosopher, Lao Tzu, once wrote: "The journey of a thousand miles begins with a single step." It is my hope this book supports you by giving you the information and insight you need on your journey as a caregiver, and more importantly, helps provide you with some peace of mind.

You are not alone.

xo – Lex

ONE

Get Your Legal Ducks in a Row

Legal Documents You Should Have & Why

I realize that you might be thinking "Legal Documents? I thought this book was about caregiving." But I assure you, there's a Zen-like peace of mind that comes from knowing that you have all the legal documents you need, because without the appropriate documents, your hands will pretty much be tied as a caregiver and there's nothing particularly peaceful about that. Also, while I'm discussing the various documents in this chapter, it might be a good idea for you to start thinking about getting your own documents together, because it's never too soon and you're never too young or too healthy to get all your own legal ducks in a row. Sadly, you never know when you might need them—as I quickly learned with my father.

Everything I know about legal documents stemmed from the fact that I knew absolutely nothing about legal documents. And the importance of having legal documents was hammered home by the fact that my father didn't have any the day he found himself in a hospital ER. At least none that anyone could find. And, for the record, having hidden legal documents is basically the same as having none at all.

I know my father had some of these documents at some point in his life because when I was about ten years old, he showed them to me, but for the life of me I don't know where they went. They just vanished. And their absence created so many problems and caused me such anxiety, all of which could have been avoided if I had just known where those suckers were.

Documents that evaporate into thin air—or cannot be found in an emergency—are of no use. Make copies, give them to people, have an attorney hold on to them, wallpaper your bathroom with them, but just make sure they are somewhere people can find them.

That said, the moment I realized something was wrong with my mother I brought her to an attorney and got all of her paperwork sorted. For obvious reasons, or for reasons that will soon become obvious, it is necessary for a person to be of sound mind when they are signing these documents.

In my experience, there are several documents you should have: a Durable Power of Attorney (POA), a Health Care Proxy, a Living Will, a Will, a Living Trust, and believe it or not, a Marriage License and Divorce papers. Depending on your financial situation, you may not need a Living Trust, but I'll get into that in a bit.

Now, at first blush, it may seem that a few of these documents do the same thing. They do mimic each other to some extent, but regardless of whether or not there is some repetition, having them will save you and your loved one a lot of heartache and headaches.

And just so you know, nothing is carved in stone, so these documents can be amended along the way if your loved one should change their mind. It's just important to get something on paper in case something should happen—which was the case with my father and his missing documents.

Durable Power of Attorney (POA)

Simply put, a Durable POA gives a designated person the legal power to make decisions for your loved one and will not expire if your loved one becomes incapacitated. A POA that is not durable could be contested if they become incapacitated, so really, what's the point of having it in the first place? For everyone's sake, just make sure this document is durable.

The scope of the POA can be either broad or narrow, depending on how much power your loved one wants to grant the person. But this should all be laid out in detail in their POA document. Generally, the decisions they are asking their POA to make on their behalf are regarding their finances and/or medical directives

It's not uncommon to break these up and give one person POA over finances, and another person POA over medical care. It's entirely up to them. Just make sure that the Medical POA includes a Health Insurance Portability and Accountability Act (HIPAA) Waiver of Authorization Form (or release form), so that their POA has access to the protected health information they may need to make educated decisions in case of an emergency. Without a HIPAA authorization form, a hospital, doctor, nurse, or any other healthcare professional will not be able to legally disclose a patient's medical information, regardless of whether someone has a POA. So again, for everyone's sake, please make sure you have a HIPAA waiver.

Something you may not know is that a power of attorney is both a document and a designation. For example: you sign a Power of Attorney (the document) making Bob your POA (designation). Therefore, Bob will be known as your POA, and as such, will also have Power of Attorney.

Don't worry, there isn't a test on this and it honestly doesn't really matter. It's just so you don't get confused if someone asks you what sounds like the same question in different ways. For instance:

Q: Do you have a POA (the document)?
A: Yes

Q: Who is the POA?
A: Bob

Q: Who has the Power of Attorney?
A: Bob

So, in this case, two thirds of the time "Bob" is the answer.

Why is a POA important? The best way I can explain this is to tell you a little story about how not having one made my life hell.

My father went to the hospital with a condition known as diverticulitis, which is a fancy name for an inflamed large intestine (or colon). He was in a lot of pain so he went to the ER where he was immediately admitted into the hospital and soon thereafter prepped for surgery to remove part of his intestines.

He was in New Jersey. I was in California. This is important to note because I wasn't there to help admit him. But because my father was conscious, he signed a piece of paper that said a family member could act on his behalf if anything went wrong during his surgery.

Initially, the surgery was a success, but within forty-eight hours, I got a call from his doctor saying he wasn't going to make it, so I jumped on a plane and flew home to be by my father's side. Once I showed up, this piece of paper my father signed that gave my family member power while he was being operated on became null and void because I was his next of kin.

"Next of kin" basically refers to the closest living blood relative. But you can see where this might get sticky, right? Let me elaborate. If the patient is married, then even though their spouse technically isn't a blood relative, they're considered the next of kin, end of story. But if the patient isn't married, their children would be considered the closest living relative. However, if they don't have children, their next of kin is a sibling, and if a sibling isn't around, then their next of kin is a niece or nephew, or maybe an aunt or uncle, or possibly even a cousin.

This gets even more complicated if they have several children, or siblings, or nieces, or whatever. Because with this next-of-kin scenario, there generally isn't any law dictating who among the children, siblings, nieces, or nephews gets to make the decisions. It's not a case where the oldest is in charge, or the biological kid has more power than the adopted one, or the favorite niece gets more say than the least favorite nephew.

Without designating a POA, it's basically up to the family to figure out if and how they're going to work together, and depending on family dynamics, that could be a total disaster. This is important to remember because without a POA, the responsibility of making decisions for you will legally fall on the next of kin—whether or not this is who you want to be making your decisions.

But back to me and my nightmare…

Theoretically, this should have been simple for me because my father wasn't married and I'm an only child, so there were no other kin anywhere to worry about. However, I had family members who, for one reason or another, felt they should be calling the shots, so they tried to take legal action to get control. That's right: family members tried to sue for the right to make medical decisions for my dad.

Nothing ever came of these lawsuits because there were simply no grounds for them. But the stress of having your father dying in a hospital while being sued by family members is something that could have been avoided if my father had designated a POA.

The POA I'm currently referring to is a Medical POA, which gives the person with the POA the power to make medical decisions on behalf of a person. But another POA that would have come in handy is a Financial POA. Even though my father had health insurance, he quickly accumulated millions of dollars in hospital debt. Millions! And that's because most health insurance only covers one hundred percent of your hospital costs for twenty days.

After those first twenty days, your insurance coverage either ends or begins to diminish until you hit a hundred days and then it completely stops altogether. After a hundred days, you either need to leave the hospital or move to a rehabilitation facility where your insurance resets and the whole hundred-day countdown begins anew.

Over a seven-month period, my father was in two hospitals and one rehab, the rehab stay being sandwiched between both hospitals. He was only in rehab for a few weeks, but both of his hospital stays exceeded a hundred days, and he was only covered one hundred percent for twenty of those days. Needless to say, the bills added up quickly and as soon as those first twenty days were up, each hospital started hounding me for payment.

As his child, I was under no legal obligation to pay his bills—though a spouse might have been—but just because they couldn't legally force me to pay didn't mean they couldn't legally harass me for payment. And they did. But there was nothing I could do because I didn't have a Financial POA.

So, one day, the hospital arranged an intervention of sorts. As we gathered around my father's hospital bed—two of his doctors, a lawyer, a psychologist, and me—his attending doctor asked him a question to determine if he was of sound mind, and because he couldn't speak, he would nod his head and point. Then the psychologist and lawyer would decide if they thought he had understood the question, and if they determined he did, his attending doctor would ask another one.

It was a long, arduous process where the end game was to get him to give me POA over his finances. But no matter how we tried, or how I begged, he wouldn't do it. Eventually, with the help of the hospital's Medicaid consultant, we devised a plan. Unfortunately, this plan entailed going to court to sue my father on the grounds that he was mentally unfit.

The idea of having to go before a judge and legally have my father declared insane was one of the lowest points of my life. In fact, I nearly had a nervous breakdown because of it. And sadly, all of this could have been easily avoided if—you guessed it—I had been granted Financial POA.

Healthcare Proxy

A Healthcare Proxy gives a chosen person the power to make health-care decisions for your loved one and is essentially the same thing as having a Medical POA—the two are interchangeable. But, regardless of what you call it, you should make sure a HIPAA Waiver (or release of Authorization Form) is included so that your loved one's Proxy can have access to their medical information should they need it.

Your loved one would designate someone as their Healthcare Proxy if they were going to split duties among people. For example, they might make one person their POA and one person their Healthcare Proxy. In this case, they would make it clear that the POA was only over finances and this would avoid any confusion as to who was responsible for what.

There are numerous reasons why someone might break up the duties between two people: one could be so no one has ultimate power, and another could be because they want everyone to feel like they're involved. A friend just made me her Healthcare Proxy and made another friend her Financial POA simply because she knew that bills stressed me out, but that I'd also "fight like hell to make sure her medical wishes were followed to a "T."

As I mentioned, because my father didn't have a POA or a Healthcare Proxy, I was automatically in charge of his medical decisions because I was his next of kin. But again, that can get messy very quickly if there is no spouse, if there is more than one child, or if there are family members who apparently want to sue you for control.

Are you beginning to understand how important these documents are?

Living Will, Advance Healthcare Directive, Do Not Resuscitate Order & Do Not Intubate Order

I've put all of these documents together because even though they are all slightly different, they all serve the same purpose—having your loved one's medical wishes fulfilled in case they are unable to advocate for themselves.

A **Living Will** is a written document where your loved one spells out their end-of-life healthcare wishes and preferences in case they should become terminally ill. This is where they establish if they want to be put on life support, if they want pain management, any religious or spiritual practices they want observed, and if they want to donate organs. Basically, anything and everything that has to do with your loved one's medical care, their body, and how they do or don't want to be kept alive can be covered in a Living Will.

An **Advance Healthcare Directive** (also known as an Advance Directive) is a document that also spells out your loved one's medical wishes in case they can't communicate them, but it isn't limited to a terminal illness. This document would express their wishes in the event they suffered a non-fatal medical condition like a stroke, or if they were diagnosed with something like dementia.

A **Do Not Resuscitate** order (also known as a DNR) is a legal document signed by your loved one and their doctor with the sole purpose of informing medical care providers about whether or not they want to be resuscitated should they go into cardiac or respiratory arrest. In other words, if they have a DNR, there will be no attempt to revive them should they have a heart attack or stop breathing.

A **Do Not Intubate** order (also known as a DNI) is essentially the same thing as a DNR except its specifically refers to not being intubated and put on a breathing device.

A Living will is an Advance Healthcare Directive, but not all Advance Healthcare Directives are Living Wills. And while a DNR and DNI could be included in their Advance Healthcare Directive or Living Will, it's always a good idea to have a new DNR and/or DNI order established each time your loved one enters a new hospital or healthcare facility just so they have it immediately accessible on file.

In my opinion, these documents might just be the most important ones of all because they determine how you live and how you die. Literally. They're that important.

What happens if your loved one doesn't have them? Then all of these decisions are left up to their POA, their Healthcare Proxy, or God forbid, their next of kin. And no one, I repeat, *no one* wants to be put in this situation—says the person who was put in this situation.

I mentioned earlier that my father had shown me some documents when I was ten years old. Well, he had also told me what they said. Which was, in essence, that he emphatically did not want to be put on life support. He felt so strongly about this that throughout the rest of his life, he would mention it to me at random times, seemingly out of nowhere. He made me promise—over and over again—that I would never, *ever,* put him on life support. And every single time, I swore I never would.

It was the biggest promise I ever broke and it still tears me apart.

My father had been in the hospital, in and out of consciousness, for about a month. I had already gotten several "your father isn't going to make it" calls and I'd flown across the country, at the drop of a hat, to be by his side every time.

Ultimately, no one was really sure what was going on. He'd have pneumonia, or a staph infection, or his kidneys were going into renal failure, and then suddenly, as if by magic, he was fine. It was during one of these "he's not going to make it, oh just kidding, he's okay" moments when everything changed forever.

I had just visited with him the day before. He was conscious, he had color in his cheeks, and he didn't look like the Stay Puft Marshmallow Man. I mention this only because, on this particular day, he wasn't any of these things—he was unconscious, pale gray, and blown up like a human water balloon.

As I stood at the foot of his hospital bed desperately trying to recognize my father, his doctor told me that if he couldn't get the fluids out of him, he would die of congestive heart failure. He believed that because my father had been on nothing but an IV for a month, the fluids he was receiving were building up in his body, causing strain on his heart. Along with the fluid retention, his body was also being flooded with toxins that weren't getting flushed out properly by his sometimes-failing kidneys, which is why he was unconscious.

Added to all of this was the fact that my father already had heart problems. He had received a quintuple bypass years ago, and he wasn't exactly a poster boy for perfect health before all this had happened. So the fact that his ticker was already impaired made this Stay Puft Marshmallow Man situation all the more dire. However, his doctor believed that if he could just pump his body full of proteins, they would naturally flush out the fluids and toxins and my father would not only deflate, he'd also wake up.

Unfortunately, this plan meant he would have to put a feeding tube in my father.

"My father made me promise to never put him on life support. Would you consider this life support?" I asked his doctor.

"No, I would consider this therapy," he responded. "We put the tube in, it does its job, and then we take it out. But it is surgery, so I will need your permission to put the tube in."

I gave him permission.

"Also, while I have him in surgery, I'd like to give him a tracheotomy (a breathing tube). He keeps pulling the oxygen tubes out of his throat and this would not only be more comfortable for him and allow his vocal cords to heal, but it would also get more oxygen into his body which will help him recover more quickly."

"Would you consider that life support?" I asked, not entirely sold on the idea.

"No, I would consider that therapy, too," his doctor responded.

"If it was your father, what would you do?" I asked.

"I'd give him the chance to live."

And there you have it. I always compare this moment to standing on the shore and watching a loved one drown. Would you throw them a life preserver or just stand there and watch them go under? I thought I was throwing my father a life preserver. Unfortunately, it turned out to be more of an anchor.

He did, in fact, deflate, but he didn't wake up. At least not for a week, but by then the therapy had been dubbed a failure and he was now, officially, on life support. Tethered to the world of the living by tubes that fed him and machines that breathed for him.

I had unintentionally broken the biggest promise I had ever made, and let me tell you, the fact that it was "unintentional" didn't make me feel any better about what I had done. Had he stayed unconscious, I would have pulled the plug and undone the horror that I had created, but the problem was that half the time he was alert. And there was no way in hell, no matter how guilty I felt, that I could pull the plug on someone who was conscious.

So what could have ended in a month by natural means had my father been allowed to go into heart failure that day, turned into a drawn out, complicated, and torturous six more months simply because he didn't have any of those documents I mentioned. If my father had made a Living Will that stated he did not want to be on life support or signed a DNI order declaring he didn't want to be intubated, the hospital never would have entertained giving him "therapy." They would have made him comfortable and he would have passed away peacefully. All his pain and drama, and millions of dollars of debt never would have happened.

Not to sound like a broken record, but can you see why these documents are so important? If you don't want to spare yourself the horror of potentially being accidentally put on life support against your will, then please spare the people you love from having to be put in that situation in the first place.

Spell it out. Let your wishes be known. Don't let your whole existence come down to a question of semantics.

A Will

A Will basically details your loved one's final wishes. It determines who gets what assets once they die, who they would like to appoint as legal guardian(s) of any minors, and what their preferences are regarding their body once they're gone.

Whereas a Living Will stipulates whether or not they'd like to donate their organs, a Will spells out what they would like to have done with their body after they die. For instance, do they want to be buried or cremated? Do they have a final resting place in mind?

Some people wish to be buried in their family plot, others want to be interred next to Grandma in a columbarium. I know someone who claims they want a Viking-like funeral, except instead of being burnt on a funeral pyre, they want to be put to blaze on a surfboard and pushed out to sea. Although, I'm pretty sure that's not legal in most states. My point is, whatever your final wishes are, your Will is where you can make them known.

Now, you may be thinking, "My loved one doesn't need a will because they don't really have anything of monetary value." Or, they may be thinking "Who cares what happens once I'm gone, I'm gone?"

I get it. A Will might not seem like an important document to some people because, let's face it, they'll be dead, so it really won't affect them. But if they have any living loved ones that they care about, then let me tell you a little story that may or may not change your mind.

As an only child, having a say in matters regarding my father's death should have been a no-brainer. There was no one else on the planet who should have had any input about this, and yet, there was. Besides telling me he didn't want to be on life support, my father had made it perfectly clear to me over the years that he wanted to be cremated and then brought on marvelous vacations to exciting, faraway places.

Considering I had royally screwed up his life support wishes, I was determined to see his cremation wishes through. But, believe it or not, a family member fought me on this. They claimed my father had told them he wanted to be in a columbarium next to his mother. A columbarium is basically a building, room, or wall in which urns are placed and then typically name plaques are hung in front of the urns to identify the remains.

The thought of my father being next to his mother was a sweet one, but considering he had never, ever, mentioned this to me, I was torn. This problem was compounded by the fact that the family member who demanded I give them my father's ashes was also one of the family members who had tried suing me for control over my father's medical care. Needless to say, in my mind, this person wasn't to be trusted.

Yet, as bad as that was, while that was going on, another family member went through my father's home sticking Post-its with their name on them all over my father's things to claim them as their own.

And when they weren't going willy-nilly with Post-its, they were sending me emails demanding to know where my father's things were.

So here I was, once again, dealing with something I never should have been dealing with, simply because my father didn't have the documentation I needed to tell them to "bug off." And while I wasn't under any obligation to grant anyone anything, I was too heartbroken and exhausted to argue about my father's belongings, so I more or less gave them whatever they wanted.

As for my father's ashes, I thought it would be nice for my dad to be near his mom, so I gave some of the ashes to my family member to have them interred with my grandmother's, and the rest I have been taking on vacation with me as promised.

So, to reiterate: if my father had a Will that stipulated what he wanted to have done with his ashes, and who exactly got what worldly possessions, I never would have been dragged through all of that drama at a time when all I wanted to do was crawl into bed and mourn my father in peace.

A Living Trust (aka a Trust)

A Living Trust allows assets to be moved around while a person is still alive, and it can come in handy for long-term care planning (which I'll get into in more detail in another chapter).

As I mentioned earlier, depending on your loved one's financial situation, they may not need a Living Trust. But if they have a lot of assets—homes, businesses, valuable possessions, investments, etc.—then they should probably have one.

While both a Trust and a Will are legal documents that technically spell out who gets what, they're different in several significant ways:

1. With a Trust, you can avoid probate. Which basically means you don't need to wait for a court to confirm the Trust before your assets are distributed.

2. Living Trusts are private, whereas a Will is made public. So if privacy is important to you and your family, then a Trust is probably the way to go.

3. You cannot set up guardianship for a minor in a Trust, but you can in a Will.

4. A Trust protects you if you should become incapacitated, but a Will does not.

5. A Trust generally takes precedence over a Will.

6. A Trust is less likely to be challenged or contested, whereas a Will is often contested.

Looking at this list, it might seem like a Trust is the better option. And again, if your loved one has a lot of assets, it might be. But a Trust costs more than a Will to set up (a Trust set up by a lawyer could cost several thousand dollars) and, unlike a Will, a Trust can get a little tricky. That's because technically, with a Trust, you no longer own your assets, the Trust does.

For example, if you have real estate that you want to leave to your children and you decide to put it in a Trust, then the Trust holds the deed, not you. This isn't a problem, per se, but if you decide to sell the real estate, it adds a level of red tape you need to go through, especially if you have someone other than yourself managing the Trust. This would also hold true for anything else held in the Trust—cars, jewelry, art, etc. It's all yours, but at the same time, it isn't.

Now, this "yours but not yours" classification can definitely come in handy if and when they are planning for their long-term care. Because the assets aren't technically theirs, it will help them and you down the line if you're considering getting them on Medicaid. But let's stick a pin in this for now, as I will get into that more in another chapter specifically about Medicaid.

My last point about a Trust is that even though you don't need a lawyer to set one up (you can get the paperwork online and set it up on your own), I would never attempt to do something as potentially complicated as setting up a Trust without some form of legal guidance. After all, the whole point of setting up a Trust is to make sure your loved ones and their assets are protected, and you're not really protecting them if you don't know what you're doing.

A Marriage License & Divorce Papers

I certainly don't need to explain what a Marriage License or Divorce Papers are, but let me explain why you need them in the context of caregiving.

After my father died, my mother, who at the point of my father's death had been divorced from him for over thirty years, said that the single most important document she had was her divorce papers. And she wasn't kidding. I'm sure if it had come down to it, it would have been easy to prove she hadn't been married to my father for decades, but because of her divorce papers, she never had to prove anything. Why would she need to prove something like that? Because my father owed millions of dollars in hospital bills and the hospitals wanted to get paid.

If, for some reason, my parents had been separated for thirty years but not divorced, my mother would have technically been responsible for my father's debt. Could she have gotten out of it? Maybe. Maybe not. Either way, it would have been costly and stressful, and who wants to go through all of that?

So if your loved one is divorced, know where those papers are and wallpaper them on the bathroom wall right alongside all their other important legal documents.

Now, a marriage license is important to have because you never know if someone is going to need it, and depending on how long they've been married, it can be hard to acquire. I found this out the hard way when I was trying to get my mother on Medicaid.

In my mind, having her divorce papers logically made her marriage license null and void. Unfortunately, while applying for Medicaid for my mother, I discovered that the Medicaid office didn't care about my logic. My guess is they had a list of documents they required, and a marriage license was on that list, right above a divorce decree.

The problem is this, marriage licenses aren't generally something someone keeps, especially after they've been divorced for thirty years, so I had to track down a copy of my parents' marriage license. This was no easy feat.

First, you need to know where the marriage took place, specifically, in what state and county, because the license will be filed by the county in which you applied for it. So, because my father was dead, and my mother had Alzheimer's, I had to figure out who was at their wedding and ask if they remembered where my parents got married in 1965. Sadly, many of their guests had passed away. Luckily, my aunt and uncle hadn't. Unfortunately, they both remembered different places. You can see how this might become difficult.

For starters, most people don't remember a wedding ceremony. They remember a wedding reception, but they often don't remember where the reception was. And, even if they remember where the reception was, that often wasn't where the couple got married, so it isn't the county where the license was filed. Needless to say, obtaining a forty-year-old marriage license can be as hard as finding a needle in a haystack.

I eventually found my parents' marriage license, but not because anyone remembered enough information for me to track it down. I actually got as far as speaking to a lovely lady in the records department of the state's capitol only to have her tell me she needed more information. I must admit, I felt pretty defeated.

However, a few weeks later, I found it stuffed in one of my father's Tom Clancy novels that had randomly appeared on the top of a large pile of books on my desk. I don't know how the book got there, or why it had their marriage license in it, but as a rule, I wouldn't count on missing documents magically showing up when you need them.

Nowadays, marriage licenses are most likely stored in a database somewhere, probably still organized by county, or at least by state. But if you got married before the advent of the internet, I would make sure a hardcopy of your marriage license is also plastered on that bathroom wall next to all the other ones, including your divorce papers, because you just never know which legal documents you're going to need. And, like I said, you can't rely on them miraculously appearing stuffed in an old book you may never think to open.

Contact Information

This sort of goes without saying, but I'm going to say it anyway: make sure you have an up-to-date contact list of all the names, numbers and email addresses of all your loved ones Legal Eagles.

Not only the name(s) of their attorney(s), but the firm's name, their paralegal(s), everyone and everything you may need to get in touch with the people you need to get in touch with. No one wants to be trying to track down these people in the middle of a crisis when emotions are running high and people often aren't thinking straight.

It not only helps your loved ones to have this information, but it will ultimately help you, too.

I'm a firm believer in the fact that when you have your ducks in a row, you often don't need your ducks at all. It's sort of like Murphy's Law, but just turned upside down and inside out—when you're prepared for the worst, the worst often doesn't happen.

Legal Last Thoughts

As I mentioned early on, I didn't have any of these documents when I needed them for my father, so the moment I suspected there was something wrong with my mother, I made sure I got everything necessary. Not only because I knew firsthand how important these documents were, but because my mother was showing signs of cognitive decline and I realized that legally she needed to understand what she was signing.

You can see why being of sound mind is important when determining who will be in charge of your finances or medical decisions, especially when you're dealing with something like a Living Will, or a DNR where you're deciding on whether or not you want to be on life support. After my own fiasco, I started hearing horror stories from friends whose parents were taken advantage of later in life by people who didn't have their best interests at heart. Fortunes were lost, heirlooms went missing, and hearts were broken.

So once again, I urge you to get all of this squared away while you and your loved one still have all your marbles intact, so to speak.

Also, while we're still on the topic of Legal Documents, I feel I should mention the importance of having a lawyer write up said documents, or at least look them over and give them their blessing. In a time when it's possible to go online and download virtually any legal form you might need, either out of convenience or a desire to save a few bucks, I implore you to reconsider. This is one area where trying to save time or money can come back and bite you or your loved ones in the ass later. Making sure these documents are ironclad is vital to their existence, because you never know when someone is going to step up and try to take control of your medical decisions or your money. Trust me on this one, I know of what I speak.

So, if you have a lawyer you regularly use for legal input, it might be wise to ask them for their two cents on the matter. If you don't, I suggest looking for either an Estate Planning Lawyer, or an Elder Law Attorney—these documents are sort of their jam.

Estate Planning Lawyers specialize in Wills and Trusts whereas Elder Law Attorneys are basically one-stop shopping when it comes to legal matters affecting aging or disabled people. Both will be able to help you with all the documents I've mentioned, but they should also be able to assist you with long-term care planning and any Medicare or Medicaid issues that come up in the future.

Every lawyer will have their own area of expertise, so you'll need to do your homework to see exactly what they do and don't do, but establishing a relationship with one now will come in handy if and when you decide to start going down the long-term care road.

Your Legal Document Checklist

- ☐ **Durable Power of Attorney (POA)**—this allows the POA to make financial and/or medical decisions on your behalf. Make sure a HIPAA Waiver of Authorization Form is included in a Medical POA.

- ☐ **Health Care Proxy**—this is the same as a Medical POA and it gives a chosen person the power to make healthcare decisions for you if you are unable to do so. Again, make sure a HIPAA Waiver of Authorization Form is included.

- ☐ **Living Will, Advance Healthcare Directive, Do Not Resuscitate Order (DNR) & Do Not Intubate Order (DNI)**—these are documents that state your medical wishes in case you are unable to advocate for yourself.

- **A Living Will** is a written document where you spell out your end-of-life healthcare wishes and preferences in case you should become terminally ill.
- **An Advance Healthcare Directive** is a document that also spells out your medical wishes in case you can't communicate them, but it isn't limited to a terminal illness.
- **A DNR** is a legal document signed by you and your doctor with the sole purpose of informing medical care providers that you do not want to be to be resuscitated should you go into cardiac or respiratory arrest.
- **A DNI** is a legal document signed by you and your doctor with the sole purpose of informing medical care providers that you do not want to intubated and put on a breathing device.

☐ **A Will**—this explains who gets what assets once you pass away.

☐ **A Living Trust**—this allows assets to be moved around while you are still alive and it can come in handy for long-term care planning.

☐ **Marriage Licenses & Divorce papers**—these are good to have just because you never know when you might need them.

☐ **Contact Information**—for all of the legal professionals you work with.

TWO

Acquire Medical Knowledge
There Is No Detail Too Tiny

While it may seem obvious that you should have all your loved one's medical information, I'm going to remind you here because it's too important to leave out: if you want to avoid unnecessary stress and anxiety, then you need your loved one's medical information!

I can't tell you how many times I was asked about my mother's blood type (though I'm still not entirely sure why), what meds she was taking, and if she had any allergies they needed to be aware of. She was AB negative, the only medication she was taking was for her thyroid, and the only thing she was allergic to was being on time. Seriously, she was always late. My father, on the other hand, was type O, took umpteen medications a day—none of which I knew the names of —was allergic to penicillin and he was always way too early to everything. Which, in my opinion, is just as annoying as being late.

I was absolutely no help to my father when he was in the hospital as far as his medical information went. I had faint memories of hospital stays and operations, but I didn't know dates, procedures, or any other pertinent facts. Fortunately, my father's long-term cardiologist was the attending doctor on call when my father went to the ER, so he already knew my father's colorful medical history and was aware of the long list of medications he took daily. It was a lucky break during an unfortunate circumstance.

That said, when the time came to tend to my mother's illness, I made sure I had all the information because I knew I couldn't count on luck again. If your loved has any sort of cognitive decline, it's imperative you start collecting all of this information while they can still be of help. And it's essential that you have the appropriate documents necessary—either a Durable Medical POA or a Health Care Proxy, both with a HIPAA waiver—so that you can collect the information you need from their medical providers.

This section is pretty self-explanatory, so I'm going to keep it short and sweet. However, don't mistake the brevity of this chapter for its significance. In order for you to effectively advocate for your loved one, it is of vital importance that you know as much information as possible.

Physicians

You should have the names, contact information, the type of medicine they practice, and the role each doctor plays in your loved one's life. This last part is important to note because some people don't have a general practitioner, they use one of their other doctors as their primary care physician. For example, I currently use my rheumatologist as my GP.

Medical Records & Results

Medical records that you should have hard copies of, or access to online, include doctors' summaries and notes, hospital discharge papers, a personal medical history—hospitalizations, surgeries, accidents, and a family medical history, if possible. Does cancer run in the family? What did their parents die from?

Ideally, you should also have information on procedures performed and test results, like blood work, urinary tests, bone density tests, mammograms, prostate tests, X-rays, CAT scans, MRIs, and ultrasound tests.

Here's an example of why all of this may come in handy...

As you are now aware, my mother had Alzheimer's. However, what you may not know is that Alzheimer's often isn't easily diagnosed. In fact, it can take years (which was the case with my mother). This is because in order to confidently diagnose a person with Alzheimer's they need to rule out virtually everything else that it could be. Thyroid. Stroke. Brain tumors. Depression. Even Lyme disease has been known to trigger dementia-like symptoms in some people. The point is, anything and everything that could cause a person to forget information and/or act erratically has to be considered and tested.

She had endless blood work done, countless MRIs and CAT scans, and umpteen psychological evaluations. And while most of those procedures were done by professionals who had my mother's medical records, there were a few instances when I had to step in and fill in the gaps with what was going on with my mother. Was information missing from her records? Or did they just not read her records thoroughly? Who knows for sure? But what I can say for certain is this: if you're advocating for someone, it's best to know what you're talking about.

Medications

You should have a list of all the current medications your loved one takes, who the prescribing doctor is, and what the dose and directions for dosage are.

Also, if you can get one of those printouts from the pharmacy that often accompanies a prescription being filled, you should keep it in your files, basically for the same reason you should have your loved one's medical records—you just never know if and when that information might come in handy.

Allergies

Know your loved one's food allergies or allergies to medications. This information will be important to know in case of an emergency.

You will also need this information if you are admitting them into a long-term care facility where, in the case of food allergies, they will need to adjust a menu or, in the case of an allergy to something like aspirin, they would need to modify their care.

Medical Bills

Keeping a file of medical bills can be helpful for a few reasons. One would be in case you are helping them with their finances, you would be able to keep track of what they owe. But mainly because it gives you a record of what doctors they are seeing and what tests or procedures are being performed.

Medical Information Last Thoughts

Apparently, the average patient only remembers about forty-nine percent of the information their doctors tell them. That percentage may decrease with the amount of information discussed, the age of the patient, and their cognitive capacity.

Needless to say, relying on accurate medical details from an aging loved one who may be suffering from cognitive decline is probably not the most effective way to acquire the medical information you need. So you may start by asking them for whatever information they can share, but you may also have to do a little detective work in their records, bills, or even calls to doctors to fill in the missing pieces.

Keep in mind that in order to play detective, you will need a Durable Medical POA or a Health Care Proxy, both with a HIPAA Waiver, so that your loved one's doctors can legally share their medical records with you.

Your Medical Information Checklist

☐ **Physicians**—You should have the names, contact information, the type of medicine they practice, and the role each doctor plays in your loved one's life.

☐ **Medical Records & Results**—This includes doctors' summaries and notes, hospital discharge papers, a personal medical history, and a family medical history, if possible. Also, try to get copies of all procedures performed and test results.

☐ **Medications**—You should have a list of all the medications your loved one takes, who the prescribing doctor is, and what the dose and directions for dosage are.

☐ **Allergies**—This could refer to food allergies or allergies to medications. This information is important to know in case of an emergency and also if you're admitting your loved one into a long-term care facility.

☐ **Medical Bills**—This will help you keep tabs on their finances, and also give you a record of what doctors they are seeing and what tests or procedures are being performed.

Become Enlightened About Insurance

Everything You Wanted to Know but Were Afraid to Ask

By the time I stepped in to help manage my parents' financial situations, both were a complete shit show. I didn't know any of it was going on until it was too late, and neither of my parents were to blame. They just both got sick and things got out of hand. Way out of hand.

But just because no one was to blame doesn't mean it wasn't awful. Because when I say "shit show," I don't use the phrase lightly. I still have panic attacks thinking about it. Hopefully, the following information can help you avoid the financial chaos I went through so that your financial experience is a far more peaceful and pleasant one than mine was.

Also, if you're wondering why I'm talking about finances in a chapter about Insurance, it's simply because the two go hand in hand. Having the proper insurance is one of the best ways I can think of to avoid most financial catastrophes. I know this from personal experience as neither of my parents had the sort of insurance that could have prevented their own financial problems.

Live and learn. Learn and teach.

I'm also going to include Life Insurance in this chapter. Traditionally, Life Insurance is something that is paid out to beneficiaries after someone has passed, but there is a version called Hybrid Life Insurance—which is life insurance and long-term care insurance rolled into one. So while regular Life Insurance won't help you care for your loved one, Hybrid Life Insurance might. Honestly, I don't have any firsthand experience with it, but I figured I'd throw it in to the mix and then you can come to your own conclusions about it. So, now let's talk insurance.

Medicare

If you're living in the United States and are over the age of sixty-five, or are younger but have certain disabilities, then you are most likely using this federal-based health insurance.

Currently, there are four primary Medicare plans: two Original Medicare Plans—Parts A and B—and two Advanced Plans—Parts C and D.

The nutshell version of what each Medicare plan covers is as follows: Part A covers hospitalization; Part B covers doctor's visits and outpatient services; Part C, often referred to as Medicare Advantage, is provided by private health insurance companies and while it primarily offers the same coverage as the Original Medicare Plans do, it often comes with extra benefits which vary depending on what insurance you buy; and Part D provides prescription drug coverage and is only offered by private insurance providers.

While Medicare does a decent job of covering your basic needs, if you end up in the hospital for seven months like my father, or if you or a loved one gets diagnosed with Alzheimer's like my mother, then Medicare alone will not be enough to help protect you from the financial hardship I encountered and that I'm trying to help you avoid.

Let's look at Alzheimer's for a moment. If you have the right Medicare plan, Medicare will cover the doctor's appointments and medication that you will need, but it will not cover any long-term care like Assisted Living or Nursing Homes. You will need something called Long-Term Care Insurance for that and we'll talk about that in a moment.

Now, if you or your loved one finds yourself in the situation that my father did, where he went into the hospital and basically never came out, then you run the risk of running out of insurance, too. Remember, if you're in the hospital, most insurance will only cover one hundred percent for twenty days, and after that, you either start footing part of the bill or, in the case with some policies, the whole bill. And unfortunately, these days, it's even more tricky to calculate costs because of all the hidden fees in health care and the potential for one of your attending doctors not being in your Network.

I can't even begin to describe the extent to which this country's healthcare system infuriates me, so let's move on to a semi-solution.

One way to protect yourself from these outrageous bills is to have Gap Insurance, also referred to as Group Supplemental Health Insurance, or Short Term Health Insurance. Medicare actually does have a version of this called Medigap which they refer to as Supplement Insurance. However, you currently cannot have Medicare Advantage and Medigap at the same time, so it's an either/or scenario. Meaning, if you're interested in going the Gap Insurance route you cannot have Medicare Plan C; in fact, it's illegal—you can only have Medicare Plans A and B. Why? I have no idea, but as I previously mentioned, this country's healthcare system infuriates me and you can add this to the long list of reasons why.

So, what is Gap Insurance?

Gap Insurance

Gap Insurance is insurance that you get to cover the gap between the period when your insurance isn't covering you and the period when it is.

Gap Insurance can help with co-payments, deductibles, and some other out-of-pocket expenses, but it may also pay for that period in the hospital when your insurance stops covering you. This bit would have really come in handy while my father was in the hospital because it would have paid his bills when his insurance started to wane after those first twenty days, and it would have allowed his insurance to restart after the hundred-day mark.

The biggest problem with Gap Insurance is that you obviously have to have it in place before you need it, and surprisingly, a lot of people don't know it exists. Even when they know about it, most people choose not to get it because it's an added expense. In these post-pandemic days, healthcare costs and out-of-pocket expenses are skyrocketing. Let's face it, they were skyrocketing before, but now they're in a whole new stratosphere.

Gap Insurance could theoretically help with this, but it's important to note that not all Gap Insurance plans cover all things, and coverage also varies by state. So if you're interested in learning more about Gap Insurance and whether or not it would work for you, you can contact your insurance agent or go to Medicare.gov and search "Medigap" to get more information.

Also, be aware that selling illegal Medigap policies has become in vogue. Because again, you are currently not allowed to be on Medicare Plan C and have Medigap, but apparently there are people out there trying to convince would-be consumers otherwise. So make sure to check with your State Insurance Department to see if the policy you are interested in is actually legit, and also go to Medicare.gov to review their list of illegal practices to watch out for.

Long-Term Care Insurance (LTCI)

Another insurance that falls into the category of, *I didn't know it existed until it was too late, but it certainly would have come in handy* is Long-Term Care Insurance (LTCI). This will reimburse you for the costs of a host of services that regular health insurance won't cover if you have a chronic medical condition, a disability, or a disorder such as Alzheimer's.

All policies are different, but usually those services include:

- Health Aid or Home Health Care, which provides assistance with bathing, grooming, taking medication, possibly light housekeeping, and other Homemaker Care tasks.
- Homemaker Care or Home Care, which helps with meal prep, laundry, cleaning, and other daily tasks seniors can no longer do for themselves.
- Respite Care for Caregivers
- Medical Equipment
- Adult Day Care
- Assisted Living
- Memory Care in Assisted Living for Alzheimer's Residents
- Nursing Home Care

What's nice about LTCI is that it generally gives you the option of how and where you receive your care. This is especially helpful if your loved one has been diagnosed with a cognitive disorder, because I can tell you from firsthand experience, trying to move a person with Alzheimer's into a new living condition can be a difficult transition for everyone. Having the option to stay at home, or somewhere familiar, can certainly take an already stressful situation and make it a little easier on the caregiver and a lot less confusing for the person suffering from cognitive decline.

But keep in mind, like most insurances, you can't wait until you need the care to buy the coverage. You won't qualify for LTCI once you've been diagnosed with a debilitating condition and most carriers won't even consider new applicants over the age of seventy-five. The average age of a person starting to buy LTCI is between the ages of fifty and sixty-five, but most people don't start using their coverage until they're in their eighties. So, considering most insurers won't accept new applicants over the age of seventy-five, it seems fair to say that waiting until your late sixties to apply might make the most sense financially, right?

Well, here's something to think about…

My mother, who was virtually never sick a day in her life, and who came from a family with no history of Alzheimer's, was diagnosed with earlyonset Alzheimer's at the age of sixty-five and it was determined, as much as it could be, that she'd probably already had the disease for ten years.

To apply for LTCI, you fill out an application, answer some health questions, submit necessary medical records, and then you're typically interviewed, either over the phone or in person, by a nurse or some other medically qualified person whose job it is to determine if you are eligible for coverage. Eligible in this case means that you don't currently need coverage and/or aren't showing any signs of needing it in the immediate future.

This means that if I had tried to get my mother LTCI when she was fifty-five—which, again, was when they determined my mother's Alzheimer's started rearing its ugly head—my mother might have been declined coverage. Now, maybe she would have, maybe she wouldn't have, who can say for sure? I certainly didn't realize she was sick at that point in her life, so maybe no one else would have either. However, I didn't know what to look for and perhaps a medically trained professional would have.

My point is that you just don't know when you're going to need it, and although the typical age of the person actually dipping into their coverage is somewhere in their eighties, you could also fall into that unexpected and unfortunate category my mom did. It's something to consider.

Now, here are some more not-so-fun-facts to add to all the other information: According to LongTermCare.gov, adults over the age of sixty-five will have a seventy percent chance of requiring some form of long-term care in their lifetime. Men typically require 2.2 years of care, while women require an average of 3.7 years—perhaps because women live longer than men, or because women are typically the caregivers for men.

Also, as I mentioned earlier, Medicare will not be covering any of your long-term care needs. It might cover a short nursing home stay or some home care with a nurse, but that's generally only when you require some sort of rehabilitation due to an accident or a medical procedure. So, if you need any of the long-term services that I mentioned above then you either need to pay for it out of pocket, buy LTCI, or get on Medicaid.

According to Genworth, a leader in financial planning and LTCI for over 145 years, the average cost in 2021 for in-home care in the United States was $61,776 for a Health Aid, and $59,488 for Homemaker Care. A private room in an Assisted Living Facility was $54,000 and a private room in a Nursing Home was $108,405. Keep in mind that these are averages, and also that Assisted Living Facilities generally charge by a sliding scale of how much care someone needs.

Because of that scale, I only paid $54,000 for the first year my mother was in Assisted Living. *Only*. After that, the cost quickly rose to $78,000 and continued to rise until it reached $106,000 a year. Needless to say, if you're paying out of pocket, which I was, you can quickly deplete your savings, a retirement fund, or a mountain of cash this way.

Okay, so maybe you're seeing the benefit of having LTCI, but you're still not entirely sold because it is an added cost. I get it. I'm all for saving money and, more importantly, for helping you save money. Just so you can see what you're potentially dealing with, here's a breakdown from the American Association for Long-Term Care Insurance (AALTCI) of the 2020 average costs for a long-term care policy:

- A single fifty-five-year-old man can expect to pay an average of $1,700 a year.
- A single fifty-five-year-old woman can expect to pay an average of $2,675 a year.
- A fifty-five-year-old couple can expect to pay an average of $3,050 a year.

Again, these are average costs, so you can probably find policies for less and definitely find policies for more. And these averages are based on the idea that the applicants are in relatively good health, so if you have some pre-existing conditions, the rates could be higher.

Also, the earlier you buy your coverage, the less it will be annually. So these average rates for a fifty-five-year-old would obviously be higher for a sixty-five-year-old. However, it's important to note that prices could go up after you buy a policy. There are no locked-in rates and prices aren't guaranteed to stay the same over your lifetime.

Now for the benefits.

The policy benefit for each policyholder is equal to the monthly benefit they choose multiplied by the duration of the policy period. For example, a long-term care policy with a $4,000 monthly benefit and a three-year benefit period would have a maximum benefit of $144,000. Some companies may have a cap limit for how many years they will pay out.

Although the numbers I've given you here will vary from case to case, you can see how having LTCI could have helped me greatly with paying my mother's bills.

Medicaid

I just wanted to pop Medicaid in here, because it is one of the insurance options you have, but I'm not going to say too much more about it, because I go into more detail in the Medicaid chapter of this book. What I do want to say about Medicaid is that I'm a big fan, and I'll tell you why.

Even though I had planned pretty well, and had enough money for most of my mom's care, it was still an exhausting, anxiety-ridden experience. I was never quite sure how much something was going to end up costing—like her Assisted Living—and I was always worried I'd run out of money before she qualified for Medicaid. And to be honest, I did. This meant I paid my mother's bills out of my own pocket for six months. So, Medicaid was a godsend for me.

Once I started the application process, the whole experience took about five months from soup to nuts. There was *a lot* of paperwork and then some meetings with a Case Manager who helped walk me through the rest of the procedures (my mother was exempt from those meetings due to her condition). Though the Case Manager was very sweet and helpful, she was overloaded, and we often played a long arduous game of phone tag just to get one question answered.

So if you decide to apply for Medicaid, have all your ducks in a row as much as possible, drop everything you're doing and answer the Case Manager's calls immediately, and above all else, be patient. That said, it was stressful, but not unbearable, and once my mother was accepted, everything changed. It felt as if a million-pound weight had been lifted off my shoulders and, for the first time in years, I felt like I could breathe again.

Suddenly, all of my mother's medical bills were covered, as was her Assisted Living and eventual Nursing Home. She was getting great medical care, she was safe and fed, and she was even getting a little monthly stipend for clothes or any other essentials she needed. I went from dreading looking in the mailbox, to getting no bills at all. And if for some reason there was a medical dispute and I got a call from one of my mother's doctor's offices, I'd just say "I'm sorry, but she's on Medicaid" and they'd apologize and leave me alone.

Medicaid was my proverbial Knight in Shining Armor and for that, I will forever be singing its praises and pushing it as a possible solution for anybody who happens to find themselves in a similar situation.

Life Insurance

Most people are familiar with the concept of Life Insurance. In fact, you can't watch TV without being bombarded by commercials reminding you that you need it and promising you peace of mind once you have it. And, truth be told, if you can afford Life Insurance, I think it's a great idea. It's a way for you to ensure your debts will get paid and your loved ones will be taken care of once you're gone. However, not all policies are created equal, so here are some things to consider if you're in the market for a Life Insurance Policy.

There are two primary types of Life Insurance—term and permanent—and they basically operate as their names suggest. A Term policy lasts a certain amount of time, or a term (usually ten to thirty years), and because of its temporary nature it is the more affordable, and it has no cash value (which is important if you or your loved one is applying for Medicaid). Whereas a Permanent policy lasts the lifetime of the policyholder, it is more expensive than a Term policy and it will eventually have a cash value as you pay into it.

There are four different types of Permanent Life Insurance: Whole Life, Universal Life, Variable Life, and Final Expense. Each of these policies will provide coverage for the life of the policyholder and each also has a savings component baked into it, which, in some cases, allows for you to borrow against the policy and/or build a nice little investment nest egg. While Final Expense, or Burial Life Insurance, falls under the category of Permanent Insurance, it basically covers what its name suggests—end-of-life expenses. Unlike Term Life Insurance, Permanent Life Insurance does have a cash value, and therefore, if you are going to be applying for Medicaid, you will most likely need to forfeit it.

Again, these insurance policies don't directly relate to caregiving, so I'm not going to go any deeper into them, but if you're interested in learning more, please speak to a Life Insurance broker. That said, I do want to say something about Hybrid Life Insurance.

Hybrid Life Insurance is essentially Permanent Life Insurance with a Long-Term Care Insurance rider attached. And while this two-for-one policy is gaining popularity with insurance buyers (I mean, who doesn't like a twofer?), it seems to be the most contentious of all the policies—which is saying a lot, because Life Insurance generally isn't controversial at all. Google "Hybrid Life Insurance" and you're sure to find articles both for it and against it. In fact, you can find articles that start out Team Hybrid and by the time they're done, they have completely talked you out of it. One of the problems is the cost: according to *Money* magazine, Hybrid Life Insurance can cost up to three times the price of Long Term Care Insurance—if you, in fact, use the Long Term Care Insurance. On the other hand, if you have Hybrid Insurance but don't use any money towards Long Term Care then that money can often be reallocated towards your Life Insurance payout. It's definitely not for those on a tight budget, but it is a Life Insurance option that can help you as a caregiver.

Your Insurance Options Checklist

☐ **Medicare**—if you're living in the United States and are over the age of sixty-five, or are younger but have certain disabilities, then you are most likely using this federal-based health insurance. It will cover some, but not all of your long-term care needs.

☐ **Gap Insurance**—additional insurance to cover the gap between the period when your insurance isn't covering you and the period when it is.

☐ **Long-Term Care Insurance**—This will reimburse you for the costs of a host of services that regular health insurance won't cover if you have a chronic medical condition, a disability, or a disorder such as Alzheimer's

☐ **Medicaid**—a federal program administered by each state which provides health coverage for eligible low-income adults, children, pregnant women, elderly adults, and people with disabilities. Along with covering healthcare costs, it will pay for Medicaid-eligible long-term care options such as assisted living facilities, nursing homes, and personal care services.

☐ **Life Insurance**—If you can afford Life Insurance it's a great idea, but it won't necessarily help with caregiving unless you have Hybrid Life Insurance. Hybrid Insurance is one part Life Insurance, one part Long-Term Care Insurance and it could be a good option if you have the money and you're on the fence about LTCI.

FOUR

Obtain Financial Insight
Money Matters Matter

Everything I learned about the importance of having a loved one's finances in order I learned the same way I did about the importance of having a loved one's legal documents squared away: out of necessity in the middle of a crisis.

I didn't have or know the information I needed for my mother when the shit hit the fan. So, once again, I found myself learning on the fly, trying to figure out what I needed and how to get it while it felt like everything around me was crumbling. Which is about as far away from zen as you can possibly get.

The moment I sensed there was something wrong with my mother—and that this issue could potentially create a financial nightmare like I had just experienced with my father—I knew I was going to start planning to get her Medicaid eligible. But even though I technically had a plan, I had none of the information I needed to implement it.

If you are reading this book to get your own ducks in a row, then great! Hopefully, you have the ability to get all your financial information together in one easy-access document or file so that when the time comes, you or your loved ones are all set. However, if you're reading this because you need help figuring out what to do for a loved one, then this might be a little more complicated. Mainly because people are weird about money.

Why? I don't know. Maybe we were raised to believe that it is rude to talk about money, or that it's nobody's business what we have. And while I believe part of this is due to the fact that we like our privacy, or that we don't want to be judged, I also believe it's because on some level—even if that person is a loved one—we just don't trust people. And this is why trying to gather financial information for a loved one can be tricky. Especially if that loved one has some sort of cognitive decline, which can often come with the added bonus of paranoia.

So what can you do? We will all have very different experiences with this based on our family dynamics. I was an only child with a single mom who I didn't realize already had moderate Alzheimer's; it was just me taking care of her. If you have siblings, a parent that was just diagnosed with Alzheimer's, and/or your parents are still married, then your experience will be very different.

That said, we still need to work together as a team regardless of how big our teams are. If you have siblings, and/or your parent has a spouse, then you need to figure out a way for everyone to get on the same page.

One way to do this is to be honest with ourselves and each other. Does one of you have a better relationship with your parent? Is one of you better with money than the others? Is someone more organized than the rest? Knowing what everyone's strengths are and playing to them will give everyone a chance to be involved in a way that best suits them, and it could help prevent resentment down the line as your parent ages.

Now, despite who is involved, the obvious first step is talking to your parent. If you have a good relationship with them and talking about money isn't verboten, then let them know that you want to gather some information about their finances so that you will be better prepared to take care of things in case of an emergency. If talking about money with your parent is a prickly topic, I have a few suggestions for how to ease into the conversation that have worked for me.

One of the best ways I know to get people talking is to ask them for advice. I don't care who they are, or if they're cognitively impaired or not, most people love giving you their opinions. Especially your parents, because no matter how old or successful you are, there is still a part of them that believes they know what's best for you. So, if you're having trouble starting a conversation with a parent about their finances, ask them for advice on yours.

For instance: "Mom, I was thinking about investing some money, where do you think is a good place to start?" Or, "Dad, someone suggested I talk to a financial advisor, do you have one you trust?" This will give you an organic opening to redirect the conversation so it becomes about them.

Another great way to start a conversation about finances is to tell them a story about somebody else's financial situation. Preferably one that didn't turn out too well so you can highlight the importance of being prepared. I know that sounds awful—like you're intentionally frightening them so that you can get what you need—so, if you have a story with a happy ending that you think will motivate them, by all means use that. My mother wasn't someone who got motivated by other people's happy endings. It was always the fear of things ending badly that put a fire under her ass. So I just used my father's story as an example of why we needed to get her ducks in a row and, for the most part, it worked.

The problem is, no matter how good your intentions are, no one wants to feel like they're losing their independence, and sometimes talking about their finances can trigger these fears. Especially if your loved one is experiencing cognitive decline. The more my mother couldn't do things for herself, the more combative she got when I tried to help her. If you're trying to have this conversation with your loved one but you keep getting pushback, just be patient, an opportunity will eventually present itself.

For me, the opportunity came when my mother became paranoid that someone was stealing her money and I offered to help her get to the bottom of it. For the record, the real story was that my mother was going to the bank almost daily and withdrawing thousands of dollars at a time. What was worse, on a few occasions (that I knew of) she lost the envelope filled with cash (God only knows about the other occasions I wasn't privy to). Then one day she looked at her statement and was shocked to see her balance, and because she didn't remember making all those withdrawals, she concluded someone else must have.

Although I was pretty certain my mother wasn't a victim of theft, I played along because I saw it as an opportunity to figure out what was going on. And then, using the story of my father's devastating financial predicament as an impetus, I offered to go through all of her financial paperwork and statements to see if there were any discrepancies. The more I played detective for her, the more I uncovered the financial mess she was in. The more I uncovered the financial mess she was in, the more I realized how sick she was.

The fact that my mother, who generally never had more than a handful of twenty dollar bills on her—ever—was now walking around with envelopes stuffed with thousands of dollars was one of the "symptoms" that led me to start seeking medical help for her. One of the other "symptoms" was that she started dating a con man. I kid you not. My completely suspicious and extremely cautious mother had met some "zillionaire" online and within two weeks she was basically inviting him to move in. Why he needed to move into her home when he apparently had several lovely, ginormous homes of his own scattered around the globe was one of the many things that made no sense to me. So I had my uncle do a background check on him and, long story short, he was a fraud.

Although I wasn't able to undo the damage she did to her own banking accounts, I was able to protect her from this swindler and safeguard the rest of her assets. Also, because I got all the financial information that I needed I was able to protect her down the line from both herself and any other fake zillionaires that might think she was an easy target.

Unfortunately, financial scams and elder fraud are the fastest growing form of elder-abuse. According to the FBI website, seniors were targeted for $1.7 billion in 2021, up seventy-four percent from the year before. Some of the scams involve lottery and sweepstake winnings, people pretending to be grandchildren calling for help and asking for money to be wired immediately, IRS calls demanding payment for back taxes, and online dating apps where Lotharios try to romance unsuspecting singles—like in the case of my mother.

Seniors are prime targets for many reasons: they are often home-owners sitting on a boatload of retirement cash; they are deemed more trusting and therefore more gullible; and they are less likely to report fraud for fear that their family might think they are unfit to care for themselves.

There are websites you can check for current Elder Fraud Scams—FBI.org has a Scams and Safety page and AARP.org has a similar Scams and Fraud page. These websites are a great source of information as they not only keep you up to date on the most common scams, but they also give you tips on how you can try and protect your loved one from becoming a target.

I didn't know about any of these websites at the time, but I knew I had to do something to protect my mother. Especially from herself. So I moved most of her money into a joint account we had set up when I had gone off to college and then I made sure she didn't have an easy way to access it. I left a limited amount of money in the account she used on a regular basis so she could use her existing debit/credit card and checkbook like she always had. It gave her the illusion of having complete financial freedom when, in fact, she was very limited. I made sure she had enough money every month to live comfortably, but not enough that if she got scammed by a grandchild she didn't have, she wouldn't be able to wire them much.

Now, keep in mind, in order for you to be able to legally do anything to help your loved one, you're going to need to have a Durable Financial Power of Attorney (POA). Otherwise, you might have all the information you need, but you won't be able to do much with it.

So, what sort of information do you need to know about your loved one's finances? I'm glad you asked!

Sources of Income

This is any money received, usually on a regular basis, from a salary, a pension, a 401k, an IRA, a trust, investments, settlements, social security, etc.

Nowadays, there are also endless ways for people to make money online. So, make sure you include this in your income search and rescue mission, otherwise it could come back to bite you.

Banking Accounts & Safe Deposit Boxes

This is every banking account your loved one may have—savings, checking, money market, certificate of deposit (CD), you name it, they all count. You will need to have all the account numbers and if they do any banking online, their usernames and passwords and any mobile banking apps they may use.

Also, if you can, get copies of any debit cards or bank cards associated with these accounts, as well as deposit and withdrawal slips.

Similarly, if your loved one has a Safe Deposit Box, you should know if there's a co-owner to the box, what its contents are, and have access to the key or have the bank issue you a copy. Also, you will need to have permission to access the box, so you either need a POA or your loved one needs to go to the bank and sign paperwork granting you access.

Insurance Policies

Again, this is every insurance policy your loved one has: health, auto, homeowners, life. If they have a policy on it, you need the information. That means the name of the insurance companies, the policy numbers, the agents, and if you can get a copy of the actual policies, even better.

In the case of life insurance, as I mentioned in the Insurance chapter, there are several different types, and it's not only important to get the policy information, but also to know what type of insurance your loved one has.

It's also important to know if any of their insurance policies have a cash value and could be seen as an asset. Just something to keep in mind when you're gathering information.

Household Debt & Documents

This pertains to anything that has to do with running the household, such as property deeds and titles, mortgage information, home equity loans, tax records, lease agreements, household bills—those kinds of things.

Property deeds and titles aside, these are usually the easiest to track down because there are often bills laying around. At least there are if your loved one still gets bills mailed to them. If your loved one gets their bills emailed to them, then it's even more important that you have all of their email accounts, usernames, and passwords noted.

Other Debt

This refers to everything else that doesn't fall under the purview of all the other financial information. This could be credit cards, auto loans, charities that get deducted automatically from bank accounts, monthly subscriptions, and the like.

Credit cards and auto loans might be something people don't want to share because they don't want to be judged for how much they're spending. So, for the sake of getting the information you need, try not to nitpick. Remember, you're trying to be helpful, not critical.

One of the ways you might be able to get the information you need if you're getting some resistance, is to offer to help them set up online banking for all their bills. This way, you'll not only have access to the information you need, but you'll also be helping them get organized.

Why You Need This

I know this is a lot to digest, but I just want you to have an idea of what you may need at some point so that you can have it ready. Nothing like scrambling around trying to track down information in the middle of a crisis to make a bad situation exponentially worse.

Now, if your loved one has a Financial Advisor, you might not need to collect any of this. However, you will need to have a POA in order for their Advisor to share any of the information you're looking for, so just keep that in mind.

If your loved one has been diagnosed with something like Alzheimer's, it's important to get all of the information you can while they can still help you get it. Generally, Alzheimer's doesn't consume them overnight, so you have time, but I believe it would be helpful to come up with a plan for their long-term care while they can still participate in it.

I say this as someone who made a long-term plan for her mother while her mother fought her the entire way. I referred to it as making plans as I was flying by the seat of my pants while my pants were on fire. I don't recommend it at all. If you can get their help and their input, I suggest you try.

If your loved one is going to need long-term care, be it in their home, your home, or some sort of assisted living or nursing home, then you are going to need some, if not all, of this information at the ready at some point. Especially if you are thinking about applying for Medicaid.

If you are considering Medicaid, then every dollar needs to be accounted for. This not only refers to assets like property and investments, but it also applies to their income, their banking accounts, and any other sources of money they may have coming in. This could also include a life insurance policy if it has a cash value, but I'll get to that in the Medicaid chapter.

Another reason you might need some of this information is so that you can protect them from elder fraud. With their banking and credit card information, you will be able to help them set up online accounts with strong passwords so that they—and you—can monitor activity. Most accounts can be set up to alert you via text or email of any suspicious or fraudulent activity.

Financial Last Thoughts

As I've mentioned, I didn't have any of this information when I needed it for either of my parents, so I understand how important it can be to get as much of the financial information you need as possible, as early as you can. Not only will it help you down the line in planning for your loved one's long-term care, it might also help you protect them from becoming a victim of an elder fraud scam.

Also, I want to pause while we're still on the topic of finances to give you my two cents on Reverse Mortgages. At first blush, it often sounds like a wonderful idea, but there are a lot of moving parts with a Reverse Mortgage and every one comes with its own set of fees. On top of fees, you are also paying interest on the money you're borrowing, and depending on how much the home is worth, there is a good chance your loved one could outlive the equity they have in their home. Meaning, they've not only lost their biggest asset, but either they, or their heirs, will owe money to the lender, and under some circumstances, the house could be foreclosed on. I considered it in my mother's situation for a brief minute, but when I started to crunch the numbers, it became crystal clear it was going to be a disaster for us. So, just keep that in mind if you're entertaining going down this path.

Your Financial Information Checklist

☐ **Sources of Income**—This is any money received, usually on a regular basis, and it can come from a salary, a pension, a 401k, an IRA, a trust, investments, settlements, social security, etc.

☐ **Banking Accounts & Safe Deposit Boxes**—This is every banking account your loved one may have: savings, checking, money-market, or certificate of deposit (CD). You will need to have all the account numbers and if they do any banking online, their usernames and passwords and any mobile banking apps they may use. You will also need information regarding the Safe Deposit Box including the key and the appropriate paperwork granting you access.

☐ **Insurance Policies**—this is every insurance policy your loved one has, including health, auto, homeowners, or life. You will need the name of the insurance companies, the policy numbers, the agents, and if you can get a copy of the actual policies, even better. In the case of life insurance, you will need to know if it has a cash value or not.

☐ **Household Debt & Documents**—This pertains to anything that has to do with running the household, such as property deeds and titles, mortgage information, home equity loans, tax records, lease agreements, household bills, etc.

☐ **Other Debt**—This refers to everything else that doesn't fall under the purview of all the other financial information. For example, credit cards, auto loans, charities that get deducted automatically from bank accounts, monthly subscriptions, etc.

☐ **Contact Information**—For all of the Insurance and Financial professionals your loved one works with.

FIVE

Open Your Mind to Medicaid

It Could Be a Lifesaver

Ultimately, all the information you'll be gathering in the other sections feeds into this one. So it's good to keep Medicaid in mind when you're going through all the other steps so that you'll collect all the information you need in order to prepare your Medicaid plan of attack, so to speak. Because there's nothing like being organized to help inspire a Zen-like vibe.

I know this from experience because my foray into Medicaid was neither organized nor zen; it happened when my father was in the hospital racking up millions of dollars of medical bills. He actually had two forms of health insurance, but one was VA insurance and because he wasn't in a VA hospital and the VA wouldn't accept him into a VA hospital, he was stuck where he was—up to his eyeballs in medical debt with no foreseeable way out.

Because the hospital wanted to get paid and neither my father nor I had millions of dollars stuffed in a mattress somewhere, the hospital came up with a plan. Get my father on Medicaid and all will be forgiven. Or, actually, get him on Medicaid and then Medicaid would work with the hospital to have them charge normal, reasonable prices for everything so that my father's bill would only be an eighth of what they were charging him, and then Medicaid would cover it.

While I was going through the paralyzing medical bill trenches with my father, I was speaking almost daily to hospital billing departments, Medicaid counselors, lawyers, and accountants—all of whom, unbeknownst to me at the time, were teaching me what could have been done to avoid the catastrophic financial situation my father had landed in. So when my mother first started exhibiting signs that something was wrong, it was almost as if I intuitively knew exactly what I had to do, except there was nothing intuitive about it. I had inadvertently gotten an accelerated degree in Medicaid.

Medicaid gets a bad rap in this country. Many people believe it's beneath them somehow to get help from the government for their healthcare. But, let me ask you this, is it beneath you to live in Paris? Or Milan? Or Madrid? Because they all provide a government-run healthcare system. In fact, most countries provide Medicaid for all of their citizens, except they don't call it Medicaid, they call it Universal Health Coverage. And no, it doesn't mean these countries are run by socialists or communists or any other kind of "ists" that we've been taught to fear; it just means these countries see the benefit of keeping their citizens healthy.

That said, I do realize there is a very real concern about becoming destitute and unfortunately, in order to qualify for Medicaid, you need to live at or under the Federal Poverty Level—and let's face it, no one willingly wants to do that. I'm going to explain some ways to help make the process less confusing and hopefully anxiety-free, and maybe even keep you from having to go broke.

Keep in mind that I am not a lawyer. I spent most of my career working in TV, but as I have mentioned, I spoke to many a lawyer while I was dealing with my father's financial debacle, so when it came time to start plotting my mother's financial course, I didn't feel the need to hire one because I already had my mother's plan seared into my brain. I did hire an attorney to write up all her legal documents, however, and I would always suggest you do that just to make sure those documents are iron-clad.

Now, in no way am I suggesting that you *don't* get a lawyer. If you can afford it, and if you're going down this path, then I'd suggest an Elder Care Attorney because this is their bailiwick. If cost is a concern, then a more affordable option might be to hire a Medicaid Specialist to help you with the application process. However, most Medicaid Specialists aren't lawyers, their main objective is to help you secure Medicaid—that's it, so if you're looking for legal advice, then a Medicaid Specialist is probably not for you. Unless, of course, they are also an Elder Care Attorney, in which case—never mind.

What is Medicaid and Why You Would Want to Be on It

Medicaid is a federal program administered by each state which provides health coverage for eligible low-income adults, children, pregnant women, elderly adults, and people with disabilities. Along with healthcare costs, it will also pay for Medicaid-eligible long-term care options such as assisted living facilities, nursing homes, and personal care services.

It is that last part that I want you to remember as I talk about Medicaid, because it's the long-term costs that will get you. So, let's stick a pin in that for now, but we'll get back to that shortly.

I was told that once upon a time all you needed to do to qualify for Medicaid was be destitute. I never checked to see if this was true, but let's just say it is for the sake of this story.

So, because being broke was theoretically the only criteria to get Medicaid, wealthy individuals would transfer all of their worldly possessions to family members, and then they'd instantly qualify. To prevent people from being rich on Monday and then Medicaid eligible on Tuesday, the government instituted what is called "a look back period" and it's exactly what it sounds like—a look back to see where all your money went and to whom.

Currently, the look-back period is sixty months (or five years) in every state but California, which is thirty months (or two and a half years.) That means in every state but California, if you had a million dollars today and gave it all away tomorrow, then five years from tomorrow, you'd be eligible for Medicaid. It's technically that simple, and yet there's absolutely nothing simple about it. Mainly because, who the hell wants to give away everything and then have to wait five years to get something in return? Also, there's a little something called living that still needs to be done between now and then, so how is that supposed to happen if you've given everything away?

Basically, there are options, most of which take some financial planning, but it means you won't be suffering while you're waiting for your eligibility. Every state has different Medicaid requirements regarding what your property assets and your monthly income limits can be in order to be eligible. Also, every state has different rules regarding what assets a spouse can retain if only one of the spouses is applying for Medicaid. Similarly, each state also has what is referred to as a Medicaid "spend down," and it is a way for an applicant who would otherwise have too much money to qualify for Medicaid to spend down their assets on Medicaid-eligible expenses like doctor's visits or on in-home care.

This is where it gets tricky to explain, because every state has vastly different rules and limits, so for this example, I'm just going to use easy made-up numbers so you can see how this all works.

Let's say you are a widow with two grown children and you have just been diagnosed with something that is going to require you to receive care for the rest of your life. You have a house worth $300,000, you get $2500 a month from social security and some other source of retirement fund, you have $10,000 in a savings account and you own your car outright. The state you live in allows you to have a house worth $400,000, but requires you to have an income of no more than $1000 a month to be eligible for Medicaid.

Because your home is below the allotted amount, you will be allowed to keep your home—if it is a primary residence and you plan on living in it during your care, returning to it from a hospital or nursing home, and/or if one of your children is going to be living in it with you to help care for you. You can also keep your car if it's going to be used for your care—say, to buy groceries and bring you to doctor's appointments. But that still means you have too many assets to qualify because you make more than the $1000 a month requirement and you have a $10,000 savings account.

This is where you'd need to spend down your assets—and you can't just gift the money away. In our example, you make $1500 more than your state's limit, so you'd need to spend $1500 a month of that money on something that qualifies for Medicaid spend down. This could be home repairs, mortgage bills, other bills, medical expenses, or home care. You need to keep copious records and all the receipts to prove you are spending every penny on qualifying things.

Also, depending on what state you live in, you may be allowed to pay a family member to be your caregiver, but it has to be done legally, with paperwork, so be careful if that's the route you decide to go. And, you would need to spend that $10,000 savings account on the same sort of Medicaid eligible things.

So, in this scenario, you could keep your home and car and still be eligible, but you couldn't keep anything else that had monetary value. But let's say you have a home worth more than what your state deems Medicaid eligible and you have investments.

Let's say your home is worth $1,000,000, you have a vacation home worth $500,000 and you have another $500,000 in investments. This may seem like a lot of money, and it is, but remember I said Medicaid might be something you consider for long-term care? Well, this is why. Currently, the average cost of a Memory Care Unit in a Nursing Home in the state I live in is about $8,000 a month. For reference, my mother lived another ten years once she was diagnosed with Alzheimer's, five of those years in Memory Care.

So, based on this $8,000 a month cost, let's go back to the example of the person with two homes worth $1,500,000 and $500,000 in investments. Using my mother as an example, if you had to pay out of pocket for a decade for their care, and five of those years they are in Memory Care at $8,000 a month (and this isn't taking into account that prices generally rise), you'd be looking at $480,000 in just room and board costs—and that doesn't include the first five years they aren't in Memory Care. Healthcare expenses like doctors and medications are not part of that. I'll pause for a second and let that sink in.

My point is, it's very easy to burn through money if someone has something like Alzheimer's. Suddenly, those two houses and half a million in investments don't seem like that much money, do they?

If you are worth millions and millions of dollars, you might be able to afford and/or stomach that sort of bill, but for most of us, health care in this country can be a nightmare. That was where I found myself and my mother, stuck somewhere between having too much and not having enough.

Let's go back to my example so I can explain what options this person might have, and then I'll tell you what I did. With two homes worth $1,500,000 and $500,000 in investments, you obviously wouldn't qualify for Medicaid, but let's say you want to because you have just been diagnosed with something that is going to require long-term care.

Remember in the Legal Documents section I mentioned something called a Living Trust? This is where that would come in handy. A Living Trust essentially makes it so you don't own your assets. You would put all your assets into a Trust and the Trust would own everything in it—your homes, your investments, your jewelry, whatever. You would appoint someone, or many someone's, as the beneficiary(s) and they would get whatever you left them once you are gone. Technically, it works like a Will, except a Will won't protect your assets.

The key to the Trust is that it protects your assets from counting as "personal" assets that you'd need to get rid of to become Medicaid eligible. However, this is also where that five-year-look-back period comes into play. You can't just put everything into a Trust and then immediately get on Medicaid—you would need to wait five years. And during that five-year period, you cannot add assets to the trust, or make donations, or give money away to family members, or go to Vegas and win a bunch of cash. You have to keep track of all your spending, accounting for all of it, or you might get penalized and your look-back period could start from scratch.

During this period of time, you'd be able to pay for living costs like food and clothes, medical expenses, and house repairs, but you need to be careful because while clothing might be considered an essential, it would be hard to argue you really needed that whole new Gucci wardrobe. I know it sounds confusing and unfair that you worked hard your entire life to acquire what you have only to be forced to hand it all over, or in the least, not have the freedom to enjoy it the way you once did or leave it to your children. But this is where having an Estate Planning Attorney or Elder Law Attorney would really come in handy.

An attorney could set up an income payment that you would receive from the Trust every month and help you create a spending plan so that you know exactly what you can and cannot do. They will also know loopholes and exemptions to help make the transition easier for you and your family. Also, if there is a spouse or a special needs child that is dependent on the funds you would otherwise be putting into a Trust, there are ways a professional could help you protect them as well.

There is another, rather drastic solution you can take with all your assets and that is to sell them all. As crazy as it sounds, that was the route I took with my mother.

At the point that I realized something was wrong with my mother, she was hemorrhaging cash. She had recently sold a second house she owned that my grandmother had lived in and she was tearing through that money at an alarming rate—over a hundred thousand dollars in less than a year. How was she doing that? Remember that story about her waltzing into the bank and withdrawing thousands of dollars at a time? That's how.

My mother's sudden interest in carrying wads of cash, coupled with her newfound desire to date con men prompted me to take her to doctors, which eventually led to her Alzheimer's diagnosis. Her strange behavior was also the impetus for my decicion to start planning for her to go on Medicaid, but before I could start planning, I had to start digging.

By the time this was going on, I had been living in California for a decade. My job in television allowed me to come home for extended periods of time, but being home for a month here and there didn't give me any insight into what was going on with her financially, so I had to dig through her finances to find out what I was dealing with.

What I ultimately discovered was that she owed hundreds of thousands of dollars in unpaid bills and hundreds of thousands of dollars more in unpaid taxes. Even though I didn't know exactly how sick she was yet, my experience with my father made it crystal clear in my mind that I was going to want to get her on Medicaid. I also knew what I was going to have to do to make that happen.

My mother didn't have any investments, so her main assets were her home and whatever was left in her bank accounts. I knew I wasn't going to be able to stay home and care for her full-time, so I calculated how much I thought I would need for her care for five years—remember the five-year look back? Then I calculated how much she owed. I determined that if I sold her house and paid off her debts, I'd have just enough money to care for her for the five years it would take before she would be Medicaid eligible.

So, why didn't I go the Trust route and protect her assets? Because I had to pay my mother's bills. I suppose I could have filed bankruptcy for her and then she could have gotten out of having to pay some of it back, but my mother had run a small business for most of my life and many of the people she owed were also small business owners and I just couldn't do that to them. I wanted them paid. So, in order to pay them I had to sell her house, and once her house was sold, there really wasn't anything left to put in a Trust. Also, I needed to get her out of her big home and closer to family, so selling her house just made sense for us on many levels.

Medicaid Waivers

So what other options do you have if, for whatever reason, you don't want to go on Medicaid?

There is something called Medicaid Waivers and they *sort of* fill in that gray area between being on Medicaid and not being on Medicaid. Medicaid waivers are often referred to as Medicaid Home and Community Based waivers or MHCB waivers, and even though they are still part of the Medicaid program, they differ in a few key ways.

First of all, the main point of a waiver is that it helps people stay in their home, or a home of a loved one, rather than having to receive care elsewhere, like in a Nursing Home. Again, each state has different requirements for becoming eligible and each state also has different waivers for different needs.

Secondly, unlike Medicaid, which is pretty much a case of once you meet the requirements you eventually get accepted, waivers generally have waiting lists. Some waiting lists might work on a first come, first served basis, while others might adhere more to a priority designation—those with the greatest need come first. Either way, each state handles their waivers differently and the waiting lists can often be long.

According to the Medicaid website, some of the services a waiver would cover are: case management, homemaker services—such as shopping, laundry and chores, home health aide, personal care, adult daycare health services, habilitation (both day and residential), and respite care to relieve a primary caregiver. Each state's waivers provide a combination of standard medical services and non-medical services, but each state differs to some degree as to what their waivers include.

A waiver could be the answer if your loved one wants to stay in their home, or maybe move into one of their children's homes, but still needs financial help for their care. An MHCB waiver would allow them to keep more of their assets than going the traditional Medicaid route, but remember, there will most likely be a waiting period, so you can't count on a waiver being a financial solution to their immediate healthcare cost problems the way you can with Medicaid.

Medicaid Final Thoughts

Medicaid has a stigma attached to it, so many people don't even consider it an option. I understand. I grew up in an affluent town and never in a million years would I have thought I'd not only be praising the virtues of Medicaid, I'd actually be one of its biggest fans. Stigma aside, I would strongly urge you to consider it because it could be a financial lifesaver.

SIX

Contemplate Long-Term Care
Not All Options Are Created Equal

Up until my parents got sick, the only experience I had with a long-term care facility was going to a nursing home every year around the holidays with my school chorus to sing Christmas carols for the residents. After my parents got sick, I became a frequent caller. For my own peace of mind, I wish I'd known more about them prior to my parents needing them, because—once again—learning while you're flying by the seat of your pants isn't the most practical way to achieve a sense of calm.

My father's experience in a long-term care facility was rather short-lived. The first hospital he was in wanted him gone because his insurance had run out and he was racking up millions of dollars in debt. Also, because they felt he was getting better and he needed to be weaned off his ventilator, which was something they didn't do.

So I flew home from Los Angeles, where I was still living, to check out a bunch of facilities the hospital had determined would be the best places for him to get the rehabilitation he needed for his lungs. I got tours of the facilities, met his potential doctors and nurses, listened to everyone's thoughts about his therapy, and even discussed what his options were financially if he needed to stay on after he recovered.

Some of the places were very institutional looking, while others were far more welcoming. In the end, I picked the facility with what I deemed was the best rehab plan and the nicest rooms. I figured if he got better and was actually conscious more than he wasn't, it would be nice for him to feel like he was in a luxury hotel room rather than a prison cell. Luckily, he loved the room. Unfortunately, he wasn't there long because he had an unforeseen life-threatening emergency: his neck exploded all over the ceiling and he had to be rushed to another hospital to save his life. I truly wish I were making that up.

Life-threatening emergency aside, once again, my experience with my father unknowingly helped pave the way for me when it came time to start looking for long-term care facilities for my mother. Although it would be a few years between hunting for a place for my father and actually moving my mother into a place of her own, I had a far better understanding of what I was looking for and, more importantly, where she would be the happiest.

By definition, a long-term care facility is a place that provides both medical and personal support to people who can no longer live independently and need assistance with daily activities such as eating, bathing, and dressing. The majority of the residents at these facilities are elderly and many of them suffer from illnesses that impact their brain function, mobility, and ability to safely care for themselves.

If you do an online search for long-term care facilities, you'll most likely get some variation of the following list: Independent Living Facilities, Assisted Living Facilities, Skilled Nursing Facilities, Nursing Homes, In-Home Care, and Continuing Care Retirement Communities.

I have personal experience with the first four, so that means I have a 66.4 percent expertise on the subject. Mathematically, I wouldn't say this makes me an expert on the topic, but experientially, it does mean I've been around the block enough to tell you what I know.

Independent Living Facility

An Independent Living Facility is designed for older adults who are still active, cognitively functioning, socially independent and generally self-sufficient. Meaning that most of the time they are capable of keeping up with daily tasks like cooking and eating, personal hygiene, light housekeeping, and monitoring their own medications.

These facilities give their residents a sense of community that they might not otherwise have living alone in a house. While everyone gets their own private, fully-equipped apartments, there are generally common areas where activities are planned and everyone can socialize. Also, there is usually some sort of director or management team onsite overseeing things.

I liken it to living in an apartment in a dorm-like situation. The apartment is yours and most residents have cars, so they can do what they want and come and go as they please. There are usually some sort of scheduled social activities every week and the residents can often be found playing cards and organizing impromptu happy hours. While management keeps a watchful eye on the residents, they don't really interfere unless they think someone's in danger.

The list of amenities differs with each facility. Some provide food and light housekeeping, some don't. Others may offer all utilities including cable, while others won't. The cost of these facilities will also vary greatly depending on where they are and how much they offer, so it's important to do your homework and know what you're looking for.

For reference, in 2009 I paid $2400 a month for a one-bedroom apartment in the suburbs of New Jersey. It was lovely, but it came with absolutely no bells and whistles. So I was also paying for my mother's cable and food. The average cost at the time for a non-Independent Living Facility one-bedroom apartment in the area was anywhere from $400 to $1400 less a month, so I was essentially paying extra for the peace of mind that came with knowing she was in a community of people who on some level would be watching out for her.

Assisted Living Facility

An Assisted Living Facility is for older adults or people with disabilities who need help with daily care to the point that living alone is no longer feasible.

There are typically different levels of care offered at an Assisted Living Facility, each with its own cost. General services usually include three meals a day, help with medications, housekeeping and laundry, transportation services, twenty-four-seven onsite staff and security, and a number of daily social and recreational activities.

The next tier of care usually includes assistance with daily care such as dressing, grooming, and help using the bathroom. Keep in mind, this is usually at an additional cost and services may be lumped together as a package, or charged individually—a la carte. Some facilities may include a Memory Care unit, which is essentially for Dementia and Alzheimer's patients. This will definitely be an additional charge and could cost nearly twice the price of the entry-level of care, if not more.

Most Assisted Living Facilities will have nurses that keep regular office hours, as well as visiting physicians specializing in all different fields of medicine who regularly make rounds at the facility and who can provide medical care to residents. Often, your loved one will start using these physicians as their primary doctors once they move in, so if they have a specific doctor that they love and trust, check to see if they can continue to use that doctor for their care.

Rooms at an Assisted Living Facility are generally a single room with a private bathroom, although some facilities may offer one-bedroom suites. They typically don't have kitchens, but may offer mini-fridges and microwaves. Rooms can be private or shared and residents are usually encouraged to bring furniture and personal items to make their space feel more homey.

Most facilities have dining rooms with daily menus that residents can choose from and daily social events like happy hour, karaoke, movie night, game night, and theme parties—all of which families are usually invited to participate in. They may also offer classes like jewelry making or arts and crafts, have lectures about anything from art to travel, and often have weekly trips to stores and local attractions. My mother's Assisted Living Facility also had a library, a beauty parlor, a business office, and a few fluffy resident pups. The main idea is to keep residents comfortable, healthy, entertained, and safe.

If an Independent Living Facility is akin to living in a dorm, then an Assisted Living Facility is more like being at camp. There are many daily activities you can choose to participate in, but you're pretty much under lock and key and they tell you when to eat, when you can leave, and where you can go.

My mother moved into her Assisted Living Facility in suburbia New Jersey in 2010. I was initially paying $4500 a month for a general level of care. However, as her needs grew, so did the cost. By the following year, I was paying over $6500 a month, and it quickly rose from there until she ended up in Memory Care at the cost of $8800 a month. Her Memory Care included room, board, and meals, but any medical assistance she needed not covered by her Medicare Insurance was paid for by me.

Remember, my intention all along was to get my mother on Medicaid, so when I was shopping around for Assisted Living Facilities I made sure to pick one that was Medicaid-eligible. This essentially means that if you pay out of pocket for a certain amount of time (each facility will have different requirements), then once the resident is eligible for Medicaid, and if the facility has a Medicaid bed available, then all the resident's bills will be covered by Medicaid.

What is a Medicaid bed? A facility can choose to get some form of government assistance in return for allocating a certain percentage of "beds" to Medicaid-eligible residents. In my mother's case, I believe her facility had allocated ten percent of its beds, which meant that if they had a hundred beds in the facility, ten had to be occupied by Medicaid-eligible residents. Which, arguably, isn't a lot.

It's important to realize that just because your loved one gets on Medicaid, it doesn't necessarily mean that a bed will be available for them. There are often waiting lists to contend with, and usually, the only way a bed opens up is for a resident to pass away, which essentially means it could be quite a long wait. So, make sure you start talking to the facility about your Medicaid goals way in advance of your loved one actually getting on Medicaid.

Also, not every Assisted Living Facility is Medicaid-eligible. So, if Medicaid is something you're entertaining down the road, make sure you find a facility that accepts it. Likewise, if your loved one already has Medicaid when you're shopping around for a facility, you'll need to make sure they have a bed available. Though this should be a lot easier for you because you'll instantly know if they have a Medicaid bed or not, rather than waiting for one to open while you're still paying exorbitant monthly bills.

Skilled Nursing Facility

A Skilled Nursing Facility is a temporary residence for patients who are undergoing some form of medically necessary rehabilitation. These facilities are often the pit stop between leaving a hospital and returning home from something like a stroke, an operation, an accident, or in the intended case of my father, being on a ventilator.

A Skilled Nursing Facility is usually a fully-staffed medical facility capable of addressing most medical situations that may arise. It's not uncommon for a Skilled Nursing Facility to be part of another facility, like a Nursing Home. Because even though a patient may have been successfully rehabilitated, it doesn't necessarily mean they are ready, or able, to go back home and care for themselves.

This was one of the many things I discussed with the facilities I went to see when I was looking for a place for my father: "What happens once he's off his ventilator, but he's still not ambulatory?" My father had been bedridden for over three months by the time I was shopping around for a Skilled Nursing Facility. He was in excruciating pain from a ginormous bedsore that was exposing his spine, the muscles in his legs had atrophied, and there were some real concerns he might not be able to walk again.

One of the things I liked about the facility I chose for my father was that once he had been successfully weaned from his ventilator, he could move to the other side of the building and receive care in a Nursing Home. After he was situated, and if he was happy, he would then have the option, if needed, to stay permanently. Of course, we never got to that point, but it was comforting to know it was there had the opportunity presented itself.

The cost of a Skilled Nursing Facility is a bit of a puzzle wrapped in a conundrum, mainly because most people are sent there from a hospital to recuperate or rehabilitate from something typically covered by insurance. Meaning, once they leave the hospital, their insurance will reset and then their first twenty days at the Skilled Nursing Home will be entirely covered. Most stays are short, so it's rare to stay past that twenty-day marker. However, if your loved one does stay longer, according to the Medicare.gov website, days twenty-one to one hundred could cost up to $194.50 a day depending on the facility and what state you live in, and then day one hundred on would be entirely at your expense.

Nursing Homes

A Nursing Home typically provides the highest level of long-term care outside of a hospital and most have skilled nurses and nurse's aides on hand around the clock. Most Nursing Homes also have a Memory Care wing for their Dementia and Alzheimer's patients. These differ from the Memory Care units at an Assisted Living Facility by the level of care they can provide.

Also, as I mentioned, some Nursing Homes are also Skilled Nursing Facilities with the main differences being the level of care and the duration of a person's stay.

At a Skilled Nursing Facility, the resident is there to receive temporary medical care while they convalesce; in a Nursing Home, the person is often there for an extended period of time because they require custodial care. Custodial care refers to non-medical assistance with the activities of daily living, such as getting in and out of bed, bathing, dressing, eating, using the toilet, and help taking medication.

While Assisted Living Facilities do offer custodial care, these facilities are generally geared toward people who can still maintain some level of daily independence. Residents in a Nursing Home are generally more dependent, requiring routine help for daily tasks.

My mother was never in the main part of a Nursing Home. She went from the beautiful Memory Care unit in her Assisted Living Facility to a sterile Memory Care unit at a Nursing Home. It was a necessary move, but a rough transition for her. She left behind a familiar space that I had decorated with many of her beloved belongings to a new and unfamiliar place where I had only a corkboard to embellish.

The cost of a Nursing Home is staggering and every state is vastly different. For instance, according to Consumer Affairs, the average cost for a Nursing Home in Alaska (the most expensive state) is $448,950 a year. *A year!* While the cost in Texas (the least expensive state) is $60,225. So if you're contemplating a Nursing Home, you're going to need to shop around and do your homework because clearly the discrepancies are vast. And, if you live in Alaska, it might be a good idea to move before you need a Nursing Home—just saying.

An important sidenote: Medicare does not cover a Nursing Home unless it's a layover from a hospital or a Skilled Nursing Facility, and even then, they will only cover one hundred percent of the cost for twenty days. But, if you or your loved one are on Medicaid, or are planning on going on Medicaid, then your cost will be nothing. Just make sure that when you're shopping around that you're looking at Nursing Homes that accept Medicaid—most of them do—but you'll want to double and triple check.

In-Home Care

In-Home Care is essentially when you stay at home and the care comes to you. The care is usually administered by a family member or a registered professional.

There are many different names and classifications for In-Home Care: Home Care, Home Health Care, Non-Medical Personal Care, and Private Duty Nursing Care, to name just a few. Each name comes with a different connotation and a list of services they provide. Some care is short-term, some long-term. Some care focuses on daily assistance around the home, while other care is more about fulfilling medical necessities.

I have known people who had help come three times a week to cook and keep them company, and others who set up a virtual hospital in their homes with round-the-clock care. The options are as limitless as the needs and the costs as varied as the reasons for staying at home.

If you have a family member or someone you know performing the care, then you obviously don't need to know what services they provide. However, if you're looking to hire a professional, then asking acquaintances or your loved one's doctors for suggestions might be a great place to start. Also, there are numerous agencies and resources online to help you find the right caregiver.

This idea of staying at home when you're aging or ill isn't a new one, but now they have a name for it: Aging in Place. An AARP survey claims that seventy-five percent of Americans over the age of fifty would prefer to stay in their homes as they age. Really, who can blame them? Many aging adults have been in their homes for years. They have an emotional connection to their homes, neighbors, and communities. And staying in their homes also gives them a sense of independence that aging, and/or a disease, often rob them of.

A friend's mother who had recently been diagnosed with Alzheimer's wanted to stay in her home specifically because she knew how to walk to her church, which she had done every day for most of her life. It gave her a sense of freedom, community, and an opportunity to exercise. My friend and her siblings decided to get her a part-time nurse, and then they divvied up the rest of the responsibilities among themselves. It was an ambitious feat of scheduling on their part as everyone worked, had families, and didn't live nearby, but it allowed their mother to stay in her home and that was more important to them than the inconvenience it caused.

I moved back east from California to care for my mother. I knew I was going to need to sell her home at some point, so I bought a condo near my family—because as an only child who traveled a lot for work, I also knew I was going to need support—and then when the time was right, I moved my mother near me.

My mother was far too independent, strong-willed, and domineering for me to just rush in and take control, so I realized I was going to have to play a long game with her. And I did. As the need to move her became apparent and the opportunity presented itself, I relocated and downsized her. Sometimes she lived with me, other times she lived alone. It was a strategic game of musical chairs where I always tried to stay one step ahead of her cognitive decline. It worked, but I must admit, it was extremely stressful.

My reason for not getting her a live-in nurse is hard to describe, mainly because you would have had to have known my mom to fully understand. She could be very charming, but she was also a force to be reckoned with and I knew, without a doubt, that she would tear through her nurses. In the end, the idea of managing rotating care-givers on a regular basis seemed far worse than the actual stress it was causing me to orchestrate all her moves.

The choice to Age in Place is a personal one. Many things factor into the decision: cost, care, the overall convenience, the personality of the person in need of care, and the ability of the family to participate in the caregiving. For some, it makes perfect sense. For others, it isn't even an option. However, I do believe that everyone knows what's truly right for them and their loved ones.

The cost of In-Home Care varies from state to state (are you sensing a pattern here?) and depends on how much assistance your loved one needs. According to a 2020 survey done by CareScout, a Genworth Financial company, the average cost for Home Care is $4481 a month. This amount is based on a forty-four-hour week and doesn't include overnight care. I just had dinner with a friend who is paying $3600 a week for Home Care for her mother who has Alzheimer's. That's $14,400 a month, which is nowhere near the national median, so again, it varies. Greatly.

Adult Day Care

Adult Day Care is somewhere older adults can go during the day to receive care and remain socially and cognitively active under the watchful supervision of professional caregivers. Although I wouldn't technically consider this a long-term care option, it can help immensely if you've decided to go the In-Home Care route.

On top of the social stimulation these centers can provide, some offer meals, medical assistance, therapeutic services, help with using the bathroom, and transportation to and from the facility. There are also centers specifically geared towards adults with Dementia or Alzheimer's, so if your loved one is cognitively impaired, these might be a perfect solution.

Attending an Adult Day Care can help thwart the feelings of isolation or loneliness that often plague aging adults who might otherwise be home alone. Remaining socially active in your golden years has proven physical, psychological, and behavioral benefits for the participants.

Another benefit of Adult Day Care is that it gives the caregiver a much-needed break to tend to their own needs: running errands, doing chores, or just catching up on rest. Adult Day Care Centers are usually open during regular business hours, so it's not uncommon for participants to be there for eight to twelve hours on any given day. This makes them a convenient option for caregivers who are continuing to work or pursuing an education, and who may not otherwise have a backup caregiver to step in while they are gone.

Depending on where you live and what services are offered, the cost can range from $25 to $100 a day. The national average for an Adult Day Care where a participant is there eight hours a day, five days a week is around $1,500 a month.

Continuing Care Retirement Communities (CCRC)

A Continuing Care Retirement Community, also known as a CCRC, is basically every long-term care option we've discussed rolled into one. It's for aging adults who want to be able to stay in the same place throughout every potential phase of their aging. CCRCs usually offer a variety of different housing options and care levels based on each person's needs.

For instance, your loved one can move into a home in the community and live independently, and then, if the need arises, move into Assisted Living, or even a Nursing Home still within the community. A friend of the family who lived in a CCRC was actually able to remain in her apartment while she received advanced medical care. They often have grocery stores, restaurants, theaters, beauty parlors, gyms, everything and anything most people could need or want.

The allure of these communities is that they provide an assortment of options in housing, care, services, and activities, so as a resident ages and their health and activity levels change, they can remain in one place and still have all their needs met. This offers them a sense of stability that they might not otherwise get, especially if they get bounced around from home to home as their health declines, like my mother unfortunately did.

It really is an awesome concept, but all that wonderful community goodness comes at a cost. Most communities charge an entrance fee which, according to the National Investment Center for Seniors Housing & Care (NIC), can range anywhere from $40,000 to $2,000,000. Of course, the price varies due to location, what type of housing option you choose, and which CCRC contract you sign. Depending on which contract you chose, that entrance fee could also cover all your medical expenses upfront. Plus, there are monthly service fees, the average cost being about $4000. So, it's definitely not the most economical long-term care solution.

I looked into this option for my mom back in 2009 because I didn't want to bounce her around if I could avoid it, but I found there were just too many variables. Her buy-in was anywhere from $250,000 to $400,000, depending on which home I chose and which contract I bought, and her service fee was going to be about $2500 a month, but that wasn't locked in and it would go up annually. I guesstimated that she would live another ten years, and if that happened, I knew I'd run out of money well before she passed away. For the record, I was right.

Long-Term Care Last Thoughts

One of the most challenging aspects of long-term care is the cost. I mean, if love and the desire to make sure everyone is happy and safe could pay the bills, we'd all be set. Unfortunately, that's not the case. The price of long-term care often means that something, somewhere, has got to give and that usually means either your money, your sanity, or both.

My intention is to help you navigate your caregiving options, not freak you out with the high price tags that often come with those options. I imagine this last section may have caused you some anxiety. I certainly know writing it has given me PTSD. So, here's a quick recap of what we've already covered and a few new tidbits of information that might help you if you're wondering, "How the hell am I supposed to pay for all of this?"

Medicare will not pay for long-term care, but Medicare Parts A, B, and C (Medicare Advantage) may pay for In-Home Care when it's medically prescribed by a doctor, carried out by a skilled medical professional, and only a temporary situation. An example would be if someone was released from a hospital or Skilled Nursing Home, but they still needed some sort of care or rehabilitation.

Depending on the state you live in, Medicaid may help cover some medical and non-medical In-Home Care costs. The Medicaid Waivers (or HCBS waivers) I mentioned earlier are specifically aimed to help with In-Home Care costs, including Adult Day Care. Just remember, most states have a limited number of waivers, and they're often distributed in a lottery-type fashion, so you can't bank on getting these the moment you need them. Another option could be one that some states offer, where Medicaid programs pay family members to be the primary caregiver to their loved one, which can help defray the costs of In-Home Care.

Long-term Care Insurance was created for this very reason—to help pay for all of your long-term care needs. Depending on your insurance coverage, and the type of care you require, it may not cover all the costs, but it will definitely pay for a large chunk of them. And, as you can see from this section, those costs can get quite chunky.

Also, if your loved one is a veteran, the VA (the U.S. Department of Veterans Affairs) offers programs that might help you pay for home care. The VA might also help you pay for Assisted Living, a Nursing Home, or Adult Day Care, but I believe you or your loved one would have to be in a VA facility. However, a VA social worker should be able to help you figure out if this might be the right path for you or your loved one.

Another option, which I must admit I do not have any experience with, is a GoFundMe campaign. According to both *Time* and *Forbes* magazines, as of 2021 $650 million dollars was raised on GoFundMe for medical campaigns. While I think this speaks volumes about how messed up our healthcare system is in the United States, I also think it says a lot about how people are willing to lend a hand, even if it's just a dollar, to help other people, often total strangers, in their time of need. If you're curious about this option, the GoFundMe website can help you start a campaign.

Reverse Mortgages are theoretically set up for this reason—for a person to be able to stay in their home while they use their home's equity for their care. I have explained why I don't like this option, but if you feel it's the right choice for you, please make sure you get a federally-insured Reverse Mortgage called a Home Equity Conversion Mortgage (HECM) which is backed by the U.S. Department of Housing and Urban Development (HUD). Because, according to the Consumer Financial Protection Bureau, Reverse Mortgage scams and foreclosures are on the rise.

Last, there are often community organizations that can help you with some of these costs. Some are state-run, some are private, and some might be churches or other places of worship, but every state has an Aging and Disability Resource Center (ADRC), that can help you figure out what resources are available to you in your community.

Your Long-Term Care Options Checklist

☐ **Independent Care Facility**—These are designed for older adults who are still active, cognitively functioning, socially independent, and generally self-sufficient.

☐ **Assisted Living Facility**—For older adults, or people with disabilities, who need help with daily care enough so that living alone is no longer feasible. Many of these facilities also have a Memory Care wing for Dementia and Alzheimer's residents.

☐ **Skilled Nursing Facility**—This is a temporary residence for patients who are undergoing some form of medically necessary rehabilitation and are often the pit stop between leaving a hospital and returning home from something like a stroke, an operation, or an accident.

☐ **Nursing Home**—This typically provides the highest level of long-term care outside of a hospital and most have skilled nurses and nurse's aides on hand around the clock. Most Nursing Homes also have a Memory Care wing for their Dementia and Alzheimer's residents.

☐ **In-Home Care**—This is essentially when you stay home and the care comes to you. Care can be short-term, or long-term, daily assistance around the home, or medical support.

☐ **Adult Day Care**—This is somewhere older adults can go during the day to receive care and remain socially and cognitively active under the watchful supervision of professional caregivers.

☐ **Continuing Care Retirement Community (CCRC)**—This is virtually every long-term care option rolled into one. It's for aging adults who want to be able to stay in the same place throughout every potential phase of their aging and health needs.

SEVEN

Learn to Improvise with Alzheimer's

The Ultimate Lesson in Going with the Flow

I want to spend a little time talking about this cruel disease. Not only because I have a decade's worth of experience with it and mention it throughout the various chapters in this book, but because it comes with its own set of challenges, one of which you can occasionally use to your advantage. Yes, *advantage*. But we'll get to that in a bit. As brutal as Alzheimer's is, going through it can actually be a very zen experience because it forces you to acknowledge you have no control. You never know from one second to the next what your loved one is going to do, say, or remember, so in order to maintain a sense of peace you must learn to be flexible and adopt an *it is what it is* sort of approach to the situation.

Also, I feel the need to remind you that I consider myself an "Accidental Caregiver." Becoming a caregiver was never on my radar, and as I have mentioned, no one in my family ever had Alzheimer's before my mother. In fact, no one in my immediate family had ever suffered any long-term debilitating illnesses until both my parents became ill, virtually back-to-back. So due to my initial lack of life experience and with absolutely no roadmap to follow, I decided to begin my foray into caregiving by drawing from the one area that I had a lot of familiarity with—working with celebrities in live television. Which, for the record, is not a very Zen-like profession.

For twenty-plus years, I worked with celebrities on award shows, morning shows, TV specials, and reality TV. So even though I had no experience with taking care of sick parents, I had tons of experience with taking care of high-profile people in a high-stress environment where you have to be prepared for the unexpected every moment. Talent arriving late to set, having hissy fits, missing their cues. When the pressure is on and the cameras are rolling, you need to be able to think on your toes and problem-solve at warp speed. Turns out, it's a lot like caregiving, minus the celebrities and cameras. So that's basically how I initially approached caring for my mother—it would be the hardest show I ever worked on with the most demanding person I've ever worked with.

Now, back to Alzheimer's…

According to the Alzheimer's Association, an estimated 6.5 million Americans over the age of sixty-five currently have Alzheimer's, and that number is projected to double in the next thirty years. According to Alzheimer's Disease International, there are over fifty-five million people worldwide currently living with the disease and every three seconds someone else in the world will develop it. The statics are staggering and terrifying. They also mean that chances are, someone you know is going to be affected by this horrible disease at some point.

The Challenges & Stages of Alzheimer's

There's a general understanding that if someone has Alzheimer's, or any form of cognitive decline, it means they are eventually going to share a common set of symptoms: difficulty remembering people, places, and events; an impaired recall of words, which will impact their ability to communicate; becoming easily confused, disoriented, and agitated; and eventually, an inability to do anything for themselves. Some people may get worse later in the day (this is known as Sundowning) and some may become restless and wander.

Each of these symptoms appears at different stages in the disease, of which there are technically three: mild (or early stage), moderate (or middle stage), and severe (or late stage). These three stages are then broken into seven more specific stages which are often referred to by number. This can get a little confusing sometimes because some people may refer to a stage as moderate, while others will say Stage Five.

My mother's doctors were often hesitant to give me a numbered stage, because I believe they didn't want to pigeon hole her into an exact box, but I was obsessed with trying to figure out where we were in the whole process, because I was trying to determine how much money I would need for her care and because I thought it would help prepare me mentally for what was coming. For the record, it didn't help with either of those things.

That said, here are the stages:

- **Stage 1: Pre-Clinical Alzheimer's**—Before symptoms appear.

- **Stage 2: Very Mild Impairment**—Basic forgetfulness associated with aging.

- **Stage 3: Mild Impairment**—Some noticeable memory loss and slight difficulty concentrating and problem solving. This is generally when household chores and paying bills start to become difficult. This Stage lasts approximately seven years.

- **Stage 4: Mild Alzheimer's**—Increased memory loss, as well as an increased difficulty with concentration, problem solving, and managing finances. Also, traveling alone to unfamiliar places might start to become challenging. They are often in denial about their symptoms and they may begin withdrawing from social interactions. This is often when a person gets diagnosed with Alzheimer's. This Stage lasts approximately two years.

- **Stage 5: Moderate Alzheimer's**—Major memory decline and decreased independence. This is when they will start to need assistance with daily activities like bathing, dressing and meal prep. They may also forget where they live, won't be able to recognize where they are or what time of day it is. This Stage lasts approximately a year and a half.

- **Stage 6: Moderate to Severe Alzheimer's**—They are experiencing severe cognitive decline and will most likely require substantial help with daily activities including going to the bathroom. Their short-term memory will be highly impaired and they may begin forgetting people's names and events from their past. This Stage lasts approximately two and a half years.

- **Stage 7: Severe Alzheimer's**—At this stage most people will have lost their ability to speak and will need assistance round the clock in virtually every aspect of their lives. This Stage also lasts approximately two and a half years.

While having a general understanding of all of this is helpful, it is important to realize that not everyone hits every symptom at the stage they are prescribed, nor will they necessarily be in that stage for the allotted amount of time given.

For instance, my mother was in Stage 4 for several years, and then basically jumped right into Stage 6 where she languished for almost four years. But even if your loved one proceeds through the disease exactly on schedule, knowing what to expect doesn't necessarily prepare you for it when it happens. And most people don't know it's happening at all until around Stage 4, and by then you're already knee deep into it.

My mother and I had a contentious relationship when I was growing up. Over the years, we both mellowed out and by the time my mother became ill, we had a loving—if somewhat complicated—relationship that is difficult to describe, but easier to illustrate.

I started to notice my mother was forgetting conversations we had just had. So one day, while we were on one of our daily phone calls, she asked me a question that I had literally just finished answering and I figured there was no time like the present to bring it up.

"Mom, you just asked me that. Don't you remember me telling you…" But before I could finish the sentence she responded with, "You're so fucking boring, I don't listen to half the shit you say. So tell me again."

Although this sort of conversation wasn't a common occurrence, it also wasn't so far out in left field for us that it caused any red flags. At least, not initially. So some of her earlier symptoms went undetected because I wrote them off as Mom just being Mom.

Another symptom I initially didn't notice was that she started hoarding things—mainly papers, but also toilets (yes, toilets), and thousands of dollars worth of home DIY materials like planks of wood and sconces that were never going to be used. The thing is, if you don't know what you are looking for, you often don't understand what you're looking at. But once you do understand what you're looking at, you suddenly start to see it everywhere. Meaning, I didn't realize she was hoarding until I did, and then it became shocking how bad it was.

My grandmother, her mother, had recently died and it really hit my mom hard. My mother's house, which had never been particularly tidy nor overtly messy, was suddenly covered in papers. Her excuse was that she needed to "file" everything away and I never questioned it. I figured she was depressed because of my grandmother, and she had gotten behind on some clerical stuff.

Then, one day, while I was home from California visiting my father in the hospital, I offered to help her get organized, and that's when I realized we were in trouble. What she was "filing" were actually old newspaper circulars from years ago heralding sales that had long passed, mixed with overdue bills, scraps of paper with doodles on them, and old forms she had used for a business she no longer had. If there was a piece of paper, regardless of what was on it, she kept it. She spent her days stapling random pieces of paper together, forming piles. Piles that she would then move around the house and go through again in the exact same manner. Every surface of her home was covered with thousands of pieces of stapled papers. So when I said earlier that I had to dig around to figure out what was going on with my mother's finances, I wasn't kidding. I literally had to go through every piece of paper to find all the bills and bank statements I was looking for.

What was almost worse than all this useless paper was the fact that she wouldn't let me throw it away. She'd become combative if I tried, and if I somehow managed to get some in the trash, she'd retrieve it when I wasn't looking. So while I was trying to fix up her house to put it on the market, my mother and her obsession with her "filing" were pushing me over the edge.

I think one of the most difficult aspects of being a caregiver to a loved one with Alzheimer's is that you're dealing with an adult who is becoming more and more childlike mentally as the days go by, but they're still in an adult form trying to maintain the independent life they once had. So every day you might be experiencing the exact same problem, obstacle, argument that you did the day before, but unlike a child who can usually learn from a situation, a person suffering from Alzheimer's can't.

Not to mention, if you agree on a solution one minute—like we're going to throw away the papers—there's no guarantee they will be okay with it ten minutes later. You often find yourself stuck in a hamster wheel, going around and around until your head is ready to explode. This is precisely when you need to get creative.

I eventually managed to get my mother to allow me to pack up her precious papers in moving boxes which we labeled "Important Documents to be Filed." I did this by making my mother think it was her idea to pack everything up. Then, I kept a few boxes with me, and told her I was moving the rest into storage. Actually, what I did was throw the rest out, but before I did, I let her watch them being loaded into the moving truck and told her she would be able to access them whenever she needed them.

Forgetfulness: Your Hidden Advantage

Remember I said there was an advantage hidden somewhere in the disease? Well, this is it. As the disease progresses, you can usually count on your loved one to forget things, especially things they aren't seeing regularly. I knew once the papers were gone, my mother wouldn't think about them again.

This forgetfulness also works in your favor for arguments, or for when they're throwing a hissy fit about something they don't want to do. Be patient, give it time, and then try again, maybe by approaching the situation differently. Chances are, with a little finessing, you'll eventually get the desired results you're looking for.

Ironically, the boxes of my mother's papers that I ended up keeping became my saving grace, and I used them to distract her for the next six years of her life. Whenever she was having a particularly difficult time adjusting to a new phase of her disease, I would open up a box of papers and sprinkle them around like fairy dust. She'd happily sort through them and "file" for days. As a publisher and editor of marketing magazines earlier in life, then a world-traveling conference speaker later, my mother's work was her life and passion. Once she got sick and was no longer working, "filing" became her new job. It gave her a sense of purpose and accomplishment, and more importantly, it kept me sane.

So my suggestion is this: take yourself out of the equation, realize they're not intentionally trying to upset you, then see what you can discover about the situation and figure out a way for both of you to get what you need.

My point in telling you about the beloved papers was to illustrate that you can often find a nugget of something helpful in the very thing that is driving you most bonkers. It's also important to realize that there is often a reason for what they are doing beyond the fact that they have Alzheimer's. They're confused, they're bored, they're scared.

Also, you, more than anyone else, know your loved one and how they are going to react to something. Even though they're disappearing, the essence of who they are is still there. So if a doctor or living facility suggests something that you know your loved one won't like, speak up. They may be the "experts" on the disease, but you're still the expert on your loved one.

For instance, when I first admitted my mom into the Assisted Living Facility and they were going over their menu of activities that they intended for my mother to participate in I knew she would have no interest in jewelry-making classes, but that she would love to sit in the library surrounded by books and listen to people give lectures. I also knew she wouldn't participate in game night, but she would definitely be all over going to the beauty parlor and getting manicures. After all, my mother was still my mother.

This was also why I was absolutely certain that she was never going to be one of those people who got lost wandering around. How was I so certain? Because my mother hated walking. Seriously. Hated it. She used to jump in her car to go halfway down the block. So one day she busted out of her Assisted Living Facility and they found her wandering in the parking lot. People said I was lucky that she had only gotten as far as the parking lot, but I knew luck had nothing to do with it. She wasn't "caught" before she managed to escape, she was caught because I'm positive she was roaming around looking for her car, which she no longer had. Now, had she still had her car, I would have been terrified, but again, I knew even Alzheimer's wasn't going to get that woman to start walking.

Every person suffering from Alzheimer's is going to have a different experience with the disease depending on what area, or lobe, of their brain is most affected. Sure, everyone more or less goes through the same stages of the disease, but each person brings their own unique traits to the experience, and that, coupled with the portion of the brain that's most damaged, means everyone will go through the stages differently. For instance, my mother never forgot me; even when she forgot my name, she called me "Her Baby." One woman in my mother's Nursing Home carried a doll and cried all the time, while another woman spent her days ripping up magazines and laughing.

It's the same with caring for a person with Alzheimer's—we all bring different attributes and baggage to the table and that, coupled with the loved one we are caring for, can make for very distinct experiences. Simply put: don't beat yourself up if you're having a really hard time being a caregiver but you see other people making it look so simple.

A lot of people can't relate to other caregivers because they aren't having the same experiences they are, or they feel guilty for being so angry all the time when other caregivers seem so cheerful. I am here to tell you, I totally understand.

At the suggestion of one of my mother's doctors, I went to an Alzheimer's support group once. Just once. I walked in as a woman was speaking about "what an honor and a privilege it was to be able to care for her mother." That was all I needed to hear. I immediately turned on my heel and walked out. While I loved my mother and there was no doubt in my mind that I would do everything within my power to care for her and make sure she was safe, there was no way in hell, considering our history, I would ever consider it an "honor" or a "privilege" to be taking care of her. Period. End of story. And the truth is, I was okay with that.

Nobody grows up dreaming about the day they get to become a caregiver to an ailing loved one. Especially if they had a complicated relationship with that person. But if you're reading this book, it tells me that despite how you feel about being a caregiver, despite the history you may have with the person you're caring for, your heart is in the right place and you're trying. And in my book—this book—that means you are just as amazing as the person who is happily doing a fabulous job of caring for their wonderful mother. So well done, you!

Alzheimer's Last Thoughts

Alzheimer's is brutal. It's one of the only diseases I know of where you can actually be mourning the loss of the person while sitting right next to them having a conversation. Technically, they are still there, and yet it's painfully clear they are gone. Sometimes it helps to remember that as difficult and scary as it is for you, it's much worse for them.

So be patient, not only with them but with yourself. If you make a mistake, lose your temper, or get pushback from your loved one, just give it time, they will eventually forget what happened and you'll get another opportunity to get it right.

A final warning when caring for someone with Alzheimer's: be careful! I won't recount every challenge I faced with my mother, including the time she tried to ambush me with a chef's knife— that's another story for another time. But I will leave you with this story: My mother's doctor told me that one of his patients stabbed her husband when he came home from work one night. She had been exhibiting signs of aggression for a while and, apparently, for one reason or another, her husband had chosen to ignore it. While uncommon, the potential for violence is there, so pay attention and be mindful of anything they might use as a weapon. Take the same precautions with knives and guns as you would with a child in the home, because it's always better to be safe than sorry.

Your Alzheimer's Stages Checklist

☐ **Stage 1: Pre-Clinical Alzheimer's**—Before symptoms appear.

☐ **Stage 2: Very Mild Impairment**—Basic forgetfulness associated with aging.

☐ **Stage 3: Mild Impairment**—Some noticeable memory loss and slight difficulty concentrating, problem-solving, doing household chores, and paying bills.

☐ **Stage 4: Mild Alzheimer's**—Increased memory loss, as well as increased difficulty with concentration, problem-solving, managing finances, and traveling alone to unfamiliar places.

☐ **Stage 5: Moderate Alzheimer's**—Major memory decline and decreased independence.

☐ **Stage 6: Moderate to Severe Alzheimer's**—Severe cognitive decline and most likely require substantial help with daily activities including going to the bathroom.

☐ **Stage 7: Severe Alzheimer's**—Most have lost their ability to speak and need assistance round the clock in virtually every aspect of their lives.

EIGHT

Make Peace with Your Grief

Because You Can't Outrun It

Grief, that horrible, heavy, painful feeling, is such a personal yet universal emotion. Just thinking about it makes my chest tighten and a prolonged sigh involuntarily escape from somewhere deep within my soul. Accepting grief as part of the caregiving process is an important step in making peace with it. It may sound simple, but it's often one of the hardest things we ever do. Grief is a complex emotion tethered to so many other emotions, anchored in our memories that are tied to the particular person, place, or thing we are grieving.

For example, the way I grieved my grandmother was very different from the way I grieved my father, which, again, was very different from the way I grieved my mother. Why? Because my life and relationships with each of them was vastly different.

My grandmother was truly one of my most favorite people in the world and I was lucky to have her for thirty-six years of my life. Even now, when I think of her, a big smile crosses my face as a million wonderful memories come flooding back: waddling around on her patio when I was a toddler, her teaching me how to ride a bike, listening to the katydids sing in the summer, and collecting pinecones together in the fall. I remember sitting at her kitchen counter talking for hours, the sound of her voice when she called my name, vacations with her, laughing together. I remember it all.

When she died, my heart shattered into a million pieces, but it was pure, unadulterated grief. It wasn't muddied by unresolved issues. It wasn't complicated by a difficult relationship. It was utter and complete heartbreak because I loved her with everything I had and now she was gone. I cried nonstop for months because I was sad and there was nothing I could do to contain it, but in a weird way, it felt good. Cathartic.

I still cry sometimes when I think about her, but it's different, the pain isn't there anymore. And in a perfect world, that's how it should be. You're sad, you hurt, you get it out, you feel better. And by better I don't necessarily mean you are done being sad, but the sad doesn't physically hurt the same way. The pain *is* the grief, and if you don't address it and process it, it doesn't go away.

So what does any of this have to do with caregiving? Everything. Unlike being a parent—which is essentially the ultimate caregiving job—when you're a caregiver to an aging or ill loved one, grief is always on the ride with us, even if we aren't aware of it. When you're caring for and raising a child, you are nurturing them with the hope that they'll ultimately go out in the world and have a wonderful, enriching life. But when you are caring for an aging or ill loved one, that life is coming to a close. There are no big dreams for bright futures with this type of caregiving, there is only the inevitable ending, and that inescapable truth means grief is never far behind.

The Five Stages of Grief

Of the hundreds of books written about grief, many follow, to some extent, the Kubler-Ross Grief Model, which states that there are five stages of grief:

1. Denial—The loss is so great and overwhelming, you initially shut down emotionally. Theoretically, this is helping you process the loss in smaller increments, but it often looks like you are trying to avoid your feelings.

2. Anger—Once you start processing your feelings, anger is often the first to the party because it's the easiest one to deal with and it offers an instant release. You might be mad at God, the person who passed, the doctors, family members—the list goes on and on.

3. Bargaining—You feel helpless and desperate for life to go back to the way it was, so you start making deals with a higher power. You might start praying for a different outcome and promising to do something in return, or you begin playing the "what if" game.

4. Depression—Now you're in the thick of it. This is when you truly begin to feel the enormity of your loss and the pain is no longer masked or subdued, it is intense.

5. Acceptance—This doesn't mean you are "okay" with your loss, it just means you accept that it happened. It can still hurt, still make you sad, but you have come to terms with the fact that your loved one is gone.

Some people argue that there are more stages, others argue that not everyone hits each stage, and some even argue that the order is wrong. But I'm not here to argue, I'm here to gently remind you to acknowledge and process your grief by sharing how I didn't acknowledge or process mine.

Grief By Any Other Name is Still Awful

I spent a year avoiding my grief about my father and a couple more years in denial that I was even grieving my mother—mainly because she was still alive and kicking. I wasn't intentionally trying to avoid grieving. I mean, I wasn't exactly running towards it with open arms, but I wasn't actively hiding from it either. I simply, or not so simply, didn't have time for it. Also, I was a bit shell-shocked.

I had watched my father slowly expire in a hospital bed for seven grueling months, flying back and forth from Los Angeles to New Jersey every other week to be by his side and advocate for his care. During that time, he teetered on the edge of life and death so often that preparing myself for the end had become part of my daily routine. Initially, I cried at the drop of a hat, but as time went on, I began suppressing my emotions. I had to be level-headed, I needed to be strong and I couldn't be any of those things and be falling apart at the same time.

Moments after my father died, I slowly felt the life force drain from my body as I became completely numb. Externally, I appeared to be functioning—people were talking to me and I seemed to be answering—but internally, I couldn't process anything I was experiencing. The pain was too deep and the loss too great. I remember leaving the hospital in a daze thinking that nothing could ever fill the ginormous hole that now took up prime real estate in my chest. And nothing did, not for a long time.

Instead of giving myself time to mourn, I immediately went back to work on one of the biggest shows I'd ever been a part of, and then I packed up my life in Los Angeles and moved back to the east coast where I jumped right back on the caregiving wagon with my mother.

Taking care of my mom while maintaining my career kept me busy round the clock, so I tried to keep my grief at bay about my father as best I could. Mainly, by not dealing with it. In my mind, my grief was like a balloon that had been blown up to maximum capacity and

I believed that it would eventually deflate on its own without any help from me, like a forgotten birthday balloon in the corner. So I went about my days pretending everything was okay. I became a master at pretending. In fact, I became so good at it that I even fooled myself. That is, until one morning when my grief literally brought me to my knees.

There was nothing particularly special about the day. It was a Saturday morning, I was in my robe checking emails as I waited for my coffee to brew when a massive force suddenly knocked the wind out of me, causing my legs to buckle. One second I was fine and standing up, the next I was on the floor, sobbing uncontrollably, gasping for air. I'm not sure how long I was there, but when the tears finally stopped and I peeled myself off the floor, I was inexplicably afraid of almost everything—leaving the house, answering the phone, talking to people.

I was in Los Angeles at the time, house-sitting for a friend while working on a show for a couple of months, and somehow—post kitchen floor episode—I still managed to go to work. But if I wasn't at work dealing with work things, I was locked in the house, irrationally fearful of having to interact with the outside world. When I had to leave, I would run to the car. If I had to get food, I would only do takeout. When friends came to check on me, I sat as far away from them as humanly possible with a blanket wrapped around me like a cloak of protection.

"I'm processing stuff," I said as they probed me for answers, quickly followed by, "and I'm not really ready to talk about it."

I wasn't lying. I was processing stuff and I wasn't ready to talk, mainly because I still wasn't entirely sure what I was processing. I mean, I was pretty sure it was Dad-related, but I didn't understand what triggered it or why I couldn't just ignore it away like I always had.

Here's the thing about grief: it really is like a blown-up balloon, except it doesn't slowly deflate over time when you pretend it's not there; it explodes. And then there's nothing you can do except what you should have done in the first place, which is to deal with it.

For me, grief manifested in many ways but depression wasn't initially one of them. First came my slow withdrawal from the outside world. I realize now it had started well before I landed on the kitchen floor, but it was happening in such small increments that it was almost undetectable. Because I was still comfortable interacting with people one on one, and in small select groups, I hadn't realized that I had ensconced myself in a protective bubble that kept most of the world at bay and gave me a false sense of security. I really thought I was doing okay, simply because I was controlling what and who had access to me, but the moment my defenses were breached, all hell broke loose.

So what breached my defenses? Moments before my collapse, I read an email from one of the talent on the TV show I was working on who claimed I was trying to starve her because she didn't like her lunch from the day before. Apparently, the salad she ordered wasn't to her liking, so she emailed me, the host of the show, and all the producers to make sure we were all aware of it. Ordinarily, this sort of thing wouldn't have pushed me over the edge, but these weren't ordinary times and clearly, I wasn't as "okay" as I thought.

Next stop on the grief train came fear, then came anger, then guilt. The fear stemmed from being constantly harassed by both family and creditors for seven months while my father was in the hospital, and I needed to process all of that before I could move on. Then I had to deal with the fact that I was apparently pissed at my father for putting me in the situation where I was under attack in the first place because he didn't have any of the necessary paperwork I needed to get everyone off my back. And finally, I had to face the guilt I felt for putting my father on life support and forgive myself for making the decisions I did. It was a lot to unpack, and it was neither easy nor pretty, but once I unraveled it all, I was finally able to grieve the loss of my father and feel heartbroken about it.

The Merriam-Webster dictionary defines grief as "deep and poignant distress caused by or as if by bereavement." *Psychology Today* describes it as "acute pain that accompanies loss." I would agree on both counts but add: it's the agonizing response to something awful we didn't want to experience in the first place that we then try to avoid because, initially, it just makes that awful thing feel ten times worse. It also makes it real.

After my father passed away, a family member wrote me a note saying that they no longer wanted to have a relationship with me because doing so reminded them that my father was gone. They contended that if I wasn't in their life, they could pretend that my father still was. They were nice about it. That is to say, besides the fact that they were telling me they never wanted to see or hear from me again, they weren't mean. And as awful as that all sounds, I totally understood their need to find peace by whatever means possible.

This perfectly illustrates how grief makes whatever you're grieving real, and it's a prime example of what being in denial looks like. As long as my family member didn't deal with their grief, or see me, my father was still alive. So to speak.

Obviously, that isn't a good way to deal with grief—but neither is doing what I did, essentially convincing myself I wasn't grieving. But grief is painful—debilitating at times—and it's completely understandable that people don't want to deal with it. Unfortunately, avoiding it not only has emotional repercussions like depression, anxiety, and collapsing on kitchen floors, it can also have physical consequences such as digestive problems, weight gain or loss, headaches, insomnia, suppressed immunity, increased inflammation, and even cardiovascular issues.

So what can you do to help alleviate your grief and protect yourself from potential health problems? I learned from personal experience that you can't ignore your grief and there are no shortcuts or detours you can take either. To paraphrase the poet Robert Frost, "The only way out is through." There are no quick fixes, no one-size-fits-all cures, and no exact timelines for how long it will take. Everyone will experience it differently and everyone will heal on their own schedule.

That said, there are things you can do which have been proven helpful with the healing process.

- For starters, acknowledge it. Acknowledge you are grieving and grant yourself the time you need to process it without judgment and without comparing your journey with anyone else's.
- Listen to your body: if you are tired, sleep; if you are sad, cry. Don't push yourself too hard and don't suppress what you are feeling.
- Take care of yourself: take your medications and vitamins, stay hydrated, eat healthy food. Your system is going through a shock and it's important to not dehydrate it, starve it, or flood it with crap.
- If you exercised before your grief set in, try to keep up that routine. If you didn't, try doing some light cardiovascular activities like going for a walk or riding a bike. Just thirty minutes of exercise can help symptoms of depression. If thirty minutes sounds daunting, try breaking it up into intervals of ten or fifteen minutes.
- Weather permitting, sit outside. Just being outside in the fresh air can boost your mood and lower your risk of depression. If you can soak in a little sunshine, even better. Sunlight has been linked to higher levels of serotonin in the brain and the release of endorphins both of which can help elevate your mood.
- Stay connected to loved ones. Don't lock yourself away. It's easy to feel like your world is shrinking so it's important that you stay connected and see people to remind you there is still life outside your grief waiting for you once you are ready.
- Do things that make you happy, or at least things that made you happy before. I believe happiness is a muscle memory,

and sometimes we just need to remind ourselves how to allow those feelings back into our lives.

- If you need professional help, get it. Talking to a therapist, a grief counselor, or a clergyperson can help you understand what you are feeling and give you much needed support while you unravel your pain.

Remember, this journey is your own to travel and only you truly know what you need or what you are feeling. So be kind to yourself and listen to your inner voice.

Grieving a Future Loss

Sometimes, you may not even realize you're grieving because no one has died. *Yet.* You would think that after collapsing on a kitchen floor, I'd have been able to spot my grief about my mother from a mile away. Not so. I completely missed it, mainly because she was still very much alive and walking around causing all kinds of trouble. I was so caught up in trying to get her diagnosed, keeping her safe, and trying to maintain my own sanity, I initially mistook my occasional crying outbursts as bouts of exhaustion. And they were, but they also weren't.

I would be doing something totally innocuous, like cooking dinner or brushing my teeth, and then suddenly burst into tears. Then, as abruptly as it started, it would stop.

One day, I was going through some of my mother's things in an attempt to organize all of the boxes that were taking over my home and I found my dog's baby teeth that my mother had kept. My mother wasn't the sentimental type, so it struck me as sweet and made me smile. But that warm fuzzy feeling quickly turned to panic as I furiously began digging through her belongings like I was on some archaeological dig, desperate to uncover proof of my mother's existence. What else had she saved? What didn't I know? Who was this woman?

I was the one who had packed all the boxes in the first place, but it had been done meticulously, with the intention of getting everything out of her home as quickly as possible so I could sell it. I didn't ruminate over every item; I'd packed everything in a logical fashion with comparable items marked for a storage unit, my home, or donation. But now, as I rifled through them, all I saw was her. Pieces of my mother on every item, in every object, throughout every box. I sat on the floor amongst her things, realizing there would be no new memories to cherish, to organize, to pack away—this was it.

Intellectually, I had understood this, but I was so focused on making sure she was okay in the moment and preoccupied with planning for her future care that I hadn't taken the time to comprehend what it all meant emotionally. But there, on the floor, in the middle of a fort of boxes filled with what was left of my mom's life, I felt the familiar pangs of grief well up deep from within my chest and I began to sob.

Alzheimer's (or Dementia of any kind) is often referred to as "the long goodbye." From the moment you suspect something is wrong with your loved one to the time they eventually succumb to this cruel disease, you have slowly lost them, piece by piece, over a protracted and agonizing period of time. Every stage comes with its own unique aspects to mourn, and every time a part of them disappears it feels like a mini-death. When they start getting lost in places they know like the back of their hand. When they can no longer do something that once brought them joy. When they begin to struggle to remember simple words. When they no longer recall anything or anyone they ever loved. It is grief by a thousand cuts and each cut breaks your heart over and over again.

Because I had run away from grieving my father, I was determined to embrace it with my mom. To not only grieve what I was losing but to grieve the loss of any possibility of a future with her. I mourned the fact that she wouldn't be at my wedding. I mourned the inside jokes we shared that I would now carry alone. I mourned every future achievement I would make that she wouldn't be a part of. If I felt it, I made sure I felt it all. I didn't run or dismiss it, I didn't cherry-pick what emotions I would allow in. I firmly planted my feet on the ground and let it all—the pain, the fear, the anger, the heartbreak—wash over me. It wasn't that I was trying to torture myself, it was that I didn't want to stop myself from feeling every ounce of it like I had with my father, only to have it sneak up on me years later and throw me on a kitchen floor.

In the end, the very end, when my mother passed away, I mourned—hard—for months. It was pure, unadulterated heartbreak like it had been with my grandmother, not the numbed-out and in-shock version I had experienced with my father. I hurt, I sobbed, but I do believe that by dealing with my grief as it surfaced along the way, I was able to diffuse the intensity of it in the end. Not that it wasn't deep or painful, but it wasn't as debilitating because it wasn't weighed down with unresolved baggage.

Grief Last Thoughts

The thing about grief is it doesn't differentiate between animal or mineral, actual or conceptional. You can just as easily mourn a place or a concept as much as you can a person. If you had to sell a family home because a loved one got sick, that can very easily feel like a death of sorts. The same holds true when the title you once held as Husband or Wife, Daughter or Son no longer exists, but rather changes in an instant to Widower, Widow, or Orphan.

You might mourn the future you will no longer have with your loved one, and the dreams you once had may have died along with them. Or you might find that the life you had before you started caring for your loved one isn't the life you can go back to once they are gone. We're so focused on our caregiving duties that sometimes we don't notice the world around us changing, and then, once we're ready to step back into our old lives, they often don't resemble the ones we left.

And we ourselves change; death has a way of doing that. No matter how hard we try, or how much we protest, we will not be the same people we were before going through the caregiving trenches. We just won't.

My point is, grief isn't always obvious and it's not always just about losing the loved one we care for. It's often about losing parts of ourselves in the process. So again, be kind to yourself. Listen to your pain, don't dismiss it. If you need to talk to a professional, do it. Don't judge yourself or your process. You need time to heal all the parts of you that are broken. And remember, as horrible as the pain of grieving may be, it is proof that we have loved. So if you can, try to infuse the pain with happy memories. I know at first that might feel like putting salt on the wound, but I do believe that love can conquer all and, by the way, salt actually helps wounds heal quicker. So there's that.

Your Grief Checklist

Here are some reminders of what you can do to heal and process your grief.

☐ Acknowledge your grief as such

☐ Listen to your body

☐ Take care of yourself

☐ Exercise

☐ Get outside and be in nature

☐ Stay connected to loved ones

☐ Do things that make you happy

☐ If you need professional help, get it

NINE

Come to Terms with Your Resentment

Psst . . . You Are Not Alone

You know that scratching sound a record makes when you drag the needle across it? It's sort of the universal sound of—hold up, wait a minute it! Some of you may be hearing that now. Here you are, reading all about how to be a more calm, peaceful, and prepared caregiver, when you hit the grief chapter and think, "Okay, I didn't see this coming, but I can go along with it…" and then, suddenly—*BAM*—you come across the word resentment and—cue the record scratch!

Maybe you don't feel any resentment about being a caregiver. (If so, perhaps you should skip this part because I'm warning you, I swear a lot in the next paragraph.) Or maybe you do resent being a caregiver but you're too ashamed to admit it. Or maybe, just maybe, you are so full of resentment that you can't even see straight. If you're part of that last group, I'm here to tell you, you are not alone.

I felt it. I felt it a lot. And while I wasn't screaming it from the rooftops, I certainly wasn't keeping it bottled up either. I swore a lot. "Fuck this. Fuck that. Fuck her." The "F" word became my mantra as I went about my day performing my caregiving duties. And thus went the first few years of caring for my mother: me dutifully doing everything I could to make sure she was cared for while leaving an unapologetic trail of F-bombs behind me. I was fortunate in the sense that I never felt the need to pretend that I didn't feel resentment. My mother and I had a complicated relationship, so I felt I had earned the right to vent if I had to. Honestly, anyone who was in my life during this period and knew our history was dropping F-bombs right alongside me.

What I find fascinating, though, is how many people don't admit they resent being a caregiver. At least, not publicly. If you try to google statistics on caregiver resentment, you'll be hard-pressed to find any, but you will find information such as 83 percent of caregivers felt it was a positive experience (according to the National Opinion Research Center), and 40 to 70 percent of caregivers suffer from feelings of depression (according to the Family Caregiver Alliance).

Now, I'm not a statistician (fun fact, my mom was!), but those two statistics seem diametrically opposed and mathematically impossible to me. Math aside, my point is: what you won't find on Google is something to the effect of *65 percent of caregivers say they absolutely resent having to be a caregiver and would rather eat glass.* Yet, many of the caregivers I talk to say that dealing with resentment is one of the hardest parts. Of course, most will immediately follow that up with something like, "But I'm happy to do it, because I love them."

And therein, I believe, lies one of the problems. We feel that if we love someone, we shouldn't resent having to take care of them. So if and when we do feel resentful, we are ashamed to admit it, and/or we feel guilty about it. But first of all, love and resentment aren't mutually exclusive. You can feel both at the same time—one doesn't cancel the other out. Also, it's possible your resentment isn't actually towards the loved one you're caring for.

Not All Resentment is Created Equal

Perhaps your resentment stems from the fact that no one else in your family is stepping up to help so the onus is on you. Therefore, you resent someone else. Or maybe it's because you feel obligated to help, but that means putting your life on hold for an indeterminable amount of time. So technically, you resent the situation. Or maybe your resentment lies in the fact that you are caring for a person who at one point wasn't particularly skilled at caring for you. In which case, you actually do resent the person you're caring for. Regardless of where it comes from, it's important to remember that resentment about your caregiver circumstances doesn't make you a bad person, it simply makes you human.

If you have family members who are physically able to help with caregiving duties and for one reason or another aren't pulling their weight, it's natural for you to feel resentment. If you have a career, or aspirations to go back to school (for instance), and all of that is now in flux while you care for your loved one, it would make sense that you would resent the situation. In these cases, it's important to communicate with the people around you—either your family, your co-workers, your boss, your professor—and explain to them what you are going through and let them know how they can help you.

Resentment can cause a downward spiral in which you begin to convince yourself that it's you against the world. "Nobody else cares. Only I can do it." And the more you do the thing that causes the resentment, the more you are convinced that you are right, you are alone. But here's the thing: very often, people don't realize what you are going through unless you tell them. Someone sees you doing a great job and they figure you don't need any help. They see you juggling caregiving and your career, and they are secretly in awe of your Super Human skills because they don't see you crumbling inside. Unless we communicate how we are feeling and what we need, we can't expect people to know.

Now, let's talk a little about the caring-for-someone-who-didn't-care-for-you part because I know that can be a major source of resentment. How do I know? I lived it. Not everyone had a *Leave it to Beaver* sort of childhood; many of us grew up in tumultuous environments and have a difficult time coming to terms with the fact that we now have to care for a parent who wasn't nurturing to us. Perhaps they were neglectful, unsupportive, or flat-out abusive. Whatever the case, faced with the dilemma of having to do for them exactly what they didn't do for you can trigger all sorts of emotions, and resentment is certainly at the top of the list.

It's helpful to remember that you don't have to do anything you aren't comfortable doing. You may feel society dictates that it is your duty to care for your sick or aging parent, but guess what? Society also dictated that your parent was supposed to care for you and how did that work out? No one but you knows what it was like growing up as you, so only you get to decide how much or how little you are capable of giving. Just you, no one else.

My mother wasn't the most maternal creature—warm and fuzzy just wasn't her thing—but if you needed a roof over your head or someone to come to your aid in an emergency, she was your gal. So, that's how I initially dealt with my resentment over being her caregiver: I gave myself permission to tend to her physical needs and keep her safe, but I decided nurturing would not be on my agenda. Ironically, and much to my surprise, when I stopped harboring all those feelings of resentment towards the situation, I realized I actually didn't mind caring for her.

Get Your Zzzz's

I have a motto I live by, which is, "Whatever helps you sleep at night." It has nothing to do with insomnia, and everything to do with your moral fiber. It's a pretty simple philosophy: if something you're about to do, or not do, is going to keep you up at night, don't do it.

The simple truth about moral fiber is that like the grain in wood, you will always get resistance when you try to cut against it. So when you're struggling in a situation, it's often because you're going against your own grain. Your grain never lies. Although, sometimes you don't realize which way your grain is going until you get there. In my case, caring for a person I love, regardless of what they did or didn't do, is part of the fiber of who I am, it's just the way my grain rolls. Now, it wasn't always easy, but I was never kept up at night pondering whether I should or shouldn't have done something while I was caring for my mother.

Resentment Last Thoughts

Here is what I am offering: if you're struggling with resentment, first stop and try to get to the bottom of what you resent. If it's something you can talk to someone about and get help with, do it. If your resentment stems from caring for someone who wasn't good at caring for you, then you need to do some soul searching to figure out exactly what you are comfortable giving them. You don't owe anyone anything, not your loved one, certainly not society, you only owe yourself to do what's right for you and, of course, whatever helps you sleep at night.

Take Care of You

Self-Care Is Not Selfish

If my adventures in caregiving taught me anything, it's that self-care is essential for creating a sense of peace and cultivating a Zen-like calm. Let's face it, if you are the primary caregiver to a loved one, or you're the chief source of financial resources for their long-term care, all of that ceases to exist if you stop functioning.

I learned this one the hard way.

According to AgingInPlace.org, over forty million people are currently caregivers to family members. Studies show that at least forty percent of all caregivers say they are stressed about their situation. Do the math—that's a whole lotta stressed caregivers! The stress of caring for a sick or aging loved one is compounded when the caregiver tries to do more than they have the time, money, or energy to manage. This is commonly referred to as "Caregiver Burnout," and it's a state of physical, emotional, mental, and financial exhaustion.

Burnout is often experienced by the caregiver, but it can also happen to the person who is orchestrating and/or paying for the care. Symptoms of burnout can include fatigue, anxiety, irritability, anger, depression, potential substance abuse, and physical ailments. While the effects are real and potentially dangerous, I've learned there are things you can do to help reduce burnout:

- Find someone you can confide in—a friend or relative—it's essential that you don't feel alone in this.
- Accept that you may need help and learn to delegate specific tasks.
- Talk to a professional or join a support group.
- Make time for yourself—alone time isn't a luxury; it's a necessity.
- Take care of your own health: eat right, take your vitamins, stay hydrated, exercise, and keep up with your own medical needs.
- Most importantly, be honest with yourself about what you can and cannot handle and acknowledge when you're in over your head.

When I first moved back to New Jersey from California to care for my mother, I was optimistic, I had a game plan and I thought I had the means to execute it. However, the daily stressors of trying to keep my mom safe while coordinating her care, coupled with the constant worry over the cost of that care, started to take its toll on me, mentally and physically.

I was in constant pain, plagued by migraines, suffering from insomnia and debilitating exhaustion, and to add insult to injury, I began experiencing recurring panic attacks. In an attempt to expunge these symptoms, I was self-medicating with dirty martinis and copious amounts of caffeine. I had hit rock bottom. Then, one day, while curled up in the fetal position in my bed praying for help—which had pretty much become part of my daily routine—I heard a voice say, "Get your shit together, Lex! You're not helping anyone like this." I was taken aback by the voice's bluntness, but I had to admit, it had a point.

I had family there to help me, people I could lean on for support, but I was truly the only one my mother had, as far as her care went, and I didn't have the luxury to fall apart. I also knew I couldn't go on the way I had been, feeling like crap, in a constant state of anxiety fueled by adrenaline and a combination of potato vodka, olives, and lattes.

So I decided I had to make a change and add some self-care practices into the whole caregiving equation. Ironically, I had pretty much been on a self-care kick and spiritual quest since I was fourteen. I was constantly on the lookout for new ways to improve my mind and calm my soul. I did yoga, I meditated, I studied Ho'oponopono, and EFT Tapping. I used Feng Shui to create positive energy in my home, and Reiki to generate positive energy in my body. I was fascinated by ancient healing modalities and blown away by new scientific findings. Yet, at the time in my life when I needed all this knowledge the most, I completely abandoned everything I knew, curled up in a ball, and let my body fall apart.

Stress is a natural part of our lives and our bodies were intrinsically designed to handle it.

Our adrenal glands release a surge of hormones, including adrenaline and cortisol. These hormones increase our heart rate, elevate our blood pressure, and give us that extra boost of energy we need to stave off a saber-toothed tiger attack—or whatever else we perceive as a danger to us in the moment. This fight-or-flight response is meant to help us cope with stress and potentially save our lives, and then it's supposed to switch off. But what happens to us when it doesn't?

Chronic stress is the feeling of being under pressure and overwhelmed for an extended period of time and anyone who is caring for a sick or aging loved one can attest to the fact that the pressure is pretty much constant. This unyielding stress can trigger skin problems, digestive disorders, autoimmune flare-ups, psychological issues, and heart disease. Stress is called "the silent killer" for a reason, but we're often too stressed out to be able to do anything about it. The problem is that being perpetually overwhelmed can cause us to become forgetful, confused. We often have difficulty concentrating and an impaired ability to problem solve. It can also lead to mental fatigue, which makes us more distracted, less motivated, and increasingly exhausted.

So essentially, the more overwhelmed you are, the less likely you are to have the energy or the mental bandwidth necessary to come up with a solution to deal with what's overwhelming you, which basically just makes you more overwhelmed.

It's a veritable catch-22, and it's why I came up with a mindful practice I call "Zen-in-Ten." Partially because I like catchy titles, but partially because the idea of spending more than ten minutes on trying to de-stress initially stressed me out. A lot. So I figured I could at least commit ten minutes a day to the idea of helping myself without taking too much time away from all the caregiving duties that stressed me out in the first place.

I was committed, but not terribly enthusiastic. The first morning I tried it, I looked myself in the mirror, pointed at my image and very matter-of-factly stated, "You got this!" I rolled my eyes and scoffed, but then I did something unexpected—I laughed. Standing there, looking at myself in the mirror, I laughed at how absolutely absurd it was that me, of all people—the one who not even twenty-four hours earlier, was rolled up in the fetal position praying for some miracle to help me with my mother and here I was now trying to be some motivating badass.

It might have been laughable, but that laugh changed everything. I mean, I wasn't instantly and magically motivated, but I was suddenly *less* unmotivated, and at the time, that was saying a lot. I set a timer for ten minutes and sat on my couch attempting to meditate as a million and one thoughts danced in my head. The next morning started with what would become a permanent part of my routine: the ol' look-yourself-in-the-mirror "You got this!" pep talk, followed by sitting on the couch for ten minutes trying to calm down.

As the days rolled on, my Zen-in-Ten would change. Some days I meditated, other days I journaled. Sometimes I did ten minutes of yoga, other times I just held my coffee cup and listed out loud everything I was grateful for. The point wasn't in what I was doing, it was simply that whatever I did, I was doing it for myself, not my mother. This is an important distinction to make as a caregiver, to carve out time where you—and only you—are your number one priority. To do something solely for yourself because it brings you peace and possibly even joy.

I began to look forward to my ten minutes in the morning, gradually fitting more Zen-in-Ten moments into random time slots throughout the day. I would turn off my phone, unplug from the outside world, and just decompress. The more I decompressed, the more I was able to see the things that caused me stress from a different perspective. The more I saw things from a different perspective, often the less stressed I became about them.

The same way being overwhelmed creates more overwhelm, being calm creates more calm. It follows the rule of quantum physics which essentially states: "Whatever you focus on you create more of."

Now, I'm not saying *Just calm down* and suddenly everything will be hunky-dory, and all your problems will magically float away. What I am offering is this: giving yourself ten minutes a day, just ten, where *you* are your one and only concern, can make all the difference in how you approach that day. And that feeds into the next day, and the next, and so on. The more you focus on the good, the less power you give the bad. The less power you give the bad, the less bad there is.

Boundaries

If caregiver burnout is a symptom of giving too much of ourselves and resentment stems from a feeling of disparity, then setting boundaries is a definite remedy for both.

Having established boundaries is, by far, one of the most important steps to self-preservation as a caregiver. They are a way we show both ourselves and others that we respect our time, our energy, and our emotional wellbeing. They help us define who we are and what we are willing and/or capable of doing as a caregiver. They establish what behaviors we will and will not accept and they help make clear what the repercussions will be if those boundaries are crossed.

Now for the bad news: setting boundaries can be one of the hardest things you'll ever do. Mainly because the people who prompt us to set boundaries—either the loved one we are caring for or the people we are sharing those caregiving duties with—often don't appreciate the fact that we've set them. So they will usually tell us we are being selfish, which can then cause us to feel guilty or ultimately question our self-worth. But let me assure you with absolute certainty: you are not selfish. In fact, I can think of nothing more selfless than caring for another being who needs us. As for your worth—nothing demonstrates a person's value and worth more than caring for another soul.

Also, I can assure you that setting boundaries and enforcing them can actually flip a switch inside your brain that will allow your feelings of self-worth to grow. The more you stand firm on your boundaries, the more your brain rewires itself to believe you are worthy of your boundaries in the first place which, in return, makes us feel more worthy.

So, now that we've established the benefits of boundaries, and the fact that you are a badass worthy of setting them, let's talk about a few ways of establishing them.

1. **Communication.** This is the key to setting healthy boundaries because you can't expect people to respect them if you don't tell people what they are in the first place. Are you sharing caregiving duties with a family member? Discuss what you're comfortable doing and what you are not. If you need a quiet hour to yourself every night before you go to bed to soak in

a bath, establish that. You can't expect people to read your mind, and then resent the fact that they didn't guess your needs. Of course, timing and presentation are everything. Find a time when you're calm and the situation isn't tense and then state your boundary in a nonconfrontational, matter-of-fact way.

2. **Saying no.** There are kind ways to say "no" without hurting people's feelings or sounding like a grump. You can be grateful: "Thank you so much for asking, but unfortunately I can't this time." You can offer them a different option: "I can't do that today, but how about tomorrow?" Or, if you feel inclined to do so, you can give them an explanation: "I've been working all day, and I'm just too tired tonight." Then again, "no" is a complete sentence, and sometimes it's important to remember that, too.

3. **Stop trying to make everyone happy.** As a caregiver, it is your responsibility to make sure your loved one is safe and cared for. However, it is not your responsibility to make them happy. Just because somebody wants something, or somebody asks you to do something, doesn't mean you have to do it. Their happiness is not your job. I repeat, their happiness is not your job. If you're doing your best and they're still not happy, that is not a reflection on you. Give yourself a pat on the back for trying and acknowledge that their mood is not part of your job description.

4. **Enforcement and consequences.** It sounds ominous, but it doesn't have to be. In fact, it's generally better to enforce your boundaries as lightheartedly as you possibly can—in a blasé, nothing-to-see-here sort of way. Your boundaries mean nothing if you draw a line in the sand and they keep stepping over

it or brushing it away. You need to enforce them and show you mean business, but you also need to be loving about it. If your family member who is supposed to be helping you with the caregiving isn't putting in their time, start making plans and tell them you're busy. If your loved one keeps walking into the bathroom while you're in the bath, install a lock. What you don't want to do is give them a pass, because a pass tells them, and you, that your boundaries don't mean anything. Even if the person you're caring for is cognitively declined and they don't remember you set certain boundaries, you enforce them anyway. You remember you set them, and these boundaries are for you just as much as they are for them.

At a couple of points in my caregiving journey, my mother lived with me in my beautiful but shoebox-sized, one-bedroom condo. The condo had exposed brick walls and fifteen-foot ceilings which were lovely but didn't help one iota when you stuck two adult humans into the space. I was cognizant of the fact that this adjustment was just as hard for my mother as it was for me, so I included her in daily activities like walking my pup or going food shopping. I made a point of taking her out to restaurants and movies a couple of times each week to keep her entertained. However, I also designated one night a week to myself when I would do my own thing, sans mom.

Initially, my mother was okay with it. In fact, I think she enjoyed having the condo to herself at first, but as time dragged on, she started getting testy. She would push her way past me as I was leaving and then follow me to my car, or if she knew where I was going, she'd show up and cause a scene. One night, while I was out on a date, she kept calling my cell to tell me I was "a selfish bitch." This is also around the time she decided to drag my family into it by calling them to say how awful I was and that she was going to disown me. But every time I came home from my night out, I'd calmly state, "I've worked hard and tonight was my night, for just me, and you getting angry about it isn't going to change anything." She'd hem and haw, but I'd never waiver and the next week we'd do the dance again.

It wasn't easy. I often felt guilty or angry or a combination of the two, but I kept going out. Not because I'm masochistic, and certainly not because I thought anything would change, but because I had worked hard and I did deserve a night out and even if my mother couldn't recognize that, I needed me to believe it.

Which brings me to my last point about boundaries: no one ever died from a guilt trip. If your loved one is trying to make you feel bad about a boundary you set, or if they've succeeded and you now feel awful about standing your ground, I'm sorry you're going through it, but I swear, you'll survive. Guilt never killed anyone. So, acknowledge the guilt, forgive yourself if you feel you are somewhat to blame, and then try practicing gratitude for everything that is good in your life. I promise you will get through this, and you will be stronger because of it.

Mindfulness

I mentioned my "Zen-in-Ten" practice earlier, and thought I'd take some time to talk about a few of those techniques in more detail here.

Nowadays, you hear a lot about mindfulness, but google the word and you can easily get overwhelmed (which is the antithesis of what being mindful is supposed to do, by the way). There are so many different takes on how many pillars (steps), elements, or principles there are to achieve mindfulness—some say two, some say nine, some say every number in between—it's easy to get confused. But no matter how you slice it, or how many pillars you may or may not have, the premise is the same: be present. Present in your mind, present in your body, present in the Now.

The Oxford English Dictionary defines anxiety as: "The state of feeling nervous or worried that something bad is going to happen."

That fear that you're in imminent danger, that you're going to run out of money, that you won't be able to meet your deadline, or that you'll never get through all the crap on your ever expanding to-do list are all very real concerns, but in reality, they probably aren't actually happening. At least not yet. Not right Now.

Anxiety has a way of hijacking our present moment and replacing it with future worst-case scenarios that often elicit a feeling of dread and render us emotionally paralyzed. Actor and humorist Will Rogers once said, "I know worrying works, because none of the stuff I worried about ever happened." While that's probably not entirely true, there is a kernel of truth to it.

Remember the episode I mentioned where I was curled up in the fetal position praying for help? Well, that whole thing started because of a fleeting thought I had first thing in the morning about my mother's escalating bills. Once that thought took hold, it quickly dragged me down a deep, dark rabbit hole where I was convinced I was going to go bankrupt and lose my home. Logically, I knew that wasn't going to happen, at least not for a couple of years, but emotionally, I was certain it already had. My point is, we get so worked up about what could happen, that we frequently lose sight of the fact that we are currently not experiencing whatever it is that we are having anxiety about. And that's essentially the key to mindfulness: being aware of where you are and what is happening around you in the present moment.

The goal is to be fully aware of your body, your surroundings, and your thoughts, in a nonjudgmental way. It's engaging all your senses and fully taking stock of the moment and checking in with reality. What are you seeing, tasting, hearing, touching? What do you know to be real in this moment?

What mindfulness is *not* is how you are feeling, because feelings have a way of making us believe them. Your feelings often come to their own conclusion about things way before you even experience them. Now, I'm not saying don't trust your feelings, but I am offering that it's probably a good idea to get into the habit of questioning them sometimes. Especially if you're having anxiety about something that isn't currently happening.

In fact, I have been known to have lengthy conversations with myself when that familiar twinge of anxiety starts to creep up. It happened a lot when I was still paying out of pocket for all of my mother's care. It generally went something like this: First, I'd sit with my anxiety, I didn't fight it, and then I'd start asking it questions: "Okay, I acknowledge you're feeling this way, but is it true, are we really in danger right now?" Then I'd wait for that little voice inside me to respond, which it always did, and it would usually start with some excuse that tried to justify why I was feeling the way I did. Once it answered, I'd listen without judgement and then I'd ask it again, "But is that true?" I'd keep asking, waiting, and listening until I'd get down to that kernel of truth, which—nine times out of ten—was that I was terrified of running out of money and then not being able to care for my mother.

As strange as it may sound, there was something about having this conversation that allowed my tightly wound brain to slowly unravel. It gave me the ability to look at my current situation as an observer, rather than a participant, which made it easier for me to acknowledge that what I was worrying about wasn't actually happening. Which then made it easier to talk myself off of the ledge I was teetering on in the first place.

If talking to your anxiety doesn't really vibe with you at the moment, but you want to try to be more in the Now, here's a simple mindfulness exercise you can try. Pick a simple task, anything, and do it so that you are completely present. For instance, wash your hands, but wash your hands acknowledging every single aspect and sensation—turning on the faucet, the feel of water on your hands, the soap between your fingers—experience it all.

Sometimes it helps to be your own commentator: "I'm washing my hands, I'm turning on the water, the water feels warm…" As silly as that may sound, taking a few minutes to be completely mindful doing something totally mindless is an easy way to start your practice of mindfulness. Then, you can move on to bigger things like having lunch or taking a hike—paying attention to every detail of the experience of an activity that you generally do absentmindedly. Slowly but surely, you'll learn to be more present in your daily activities, which will come in handy when you're overwhelmed by your caregiving duties and you need to completely disconnect but you can't totally disappear.

Meditation

While meditation is technically a form of mindfulness, and vice versa, there are a few significant differences between the two. Mindfulness is a way to experience and connect with the world around you, while meditation is a practice you do to go inward and connect with yourself. Mindfulness is a state of being fully present in the moment and can be done anywhere at any time, while meditation is a formal practice which is done with the intention of expanding your consciousness and calming your mind. It's one of my go-to Zen-in-Ten practices for that very reason.

Just like mindfulness, there are many types of meditation. The website of meditation guru Deepak Chopra, chopra.com, gives examples of five different types of meditation—breath-awareness meditation, loving-kindness meditation, mantra-based meditation, visualization meditation, and guided meditation. But you can easily find more variations online.

I started my meditation practice in my teens with guided meditation, one of the easiest ways to dip your toe into the meditation waters because, as the name suggests, you have someone guiding you through the whole experience, which means your brain is less likely to jump around like a crazy monkey (also known as Monkey Mind—yes, that's a real term). Years later, when my father passed, I started practicing Transcendental Meditation (TM), a practice where silently repeating a mantra can guide you into a deep, meditative state.

When I hit rock bottom while caring for my mother, I found meditation to be the number one way to quell my anxiety. I also found it incredibly difficult at first because my mind was bouncing around from worrying about my mom, to thinking about work, to stressing about money. But because I had experience with meditation being helpful in the past, I kept at it every day and within a few weeks, I started to notice a calm wash over me. It wasn't that I stopped thinking about all the things I was worried about, but they didn't have the same paralyzing impact on me.

If you're having trouble getting started, here's a simple technique that might help you begin to calm your mind. Find somewhere quiet where you can relax. Get comfortable, I suggest sitting, but if lying down feels right to you, follow your gut. Slowly take three big, deep breaths—in through your nose, out through your mouth—and then set an intention to create a few moments of peace for yourself.

Now pick a word, I would suggest something positive like the word "Love" or the phrase "I am Peace." Slowly repeat the word/phrase over and over, syncing it with your breath (which you can now do however feels most natural). Pay attention to your breathing, acknowledge any thoughts that pop into your head, but don't judge them. If something negative comes up, thank it for its opinion and let it go. Try doing this for five minutes at first, and then work up to ten. Don't stress out about it if it initially doesn't come easily. Ironically, finding peace can often be extremely aggravating at first. But remember, every minute you're not stressing out is a win for your nervous system, and a win for you as a caregiver.

Journaling

Now, journaling may not sound as mystical as mindfulness or meditation, but it can certainly be as magical, and like the other Zen-in-Ten practices I've mentioned, it also has mental and physical benefits.

According to a research article written by Karen A. Baikie and Kay Wilhelm on the "Emotional and physical health benefits of expressive writing," the long-term benefits of expressive writing (such as journaling) about a traumatic experience not only helps reduce stress, it can also improve immune function, lower blood pressure, improve liver function, and improve overall psychological well-being. You might be thinking, "Hold the phone! I understand how journaling might help reduce stress, but improve liver function?" Here's my theory on that. In Acupuncture and Eastern Medicine, the emotion associated with the liver is anger, so if you're journaling and releasing all that pent-up anger onto your pages, your liver will reap the benefits of getting a break from processing all that negative energy. Again, I'm not a doctor, and this is just a theory, but it makes sense to me.

At first blush, journaling might not seem like a very Zen practice because we've come to believe that Zenning-out is about sitting in a lotus position (cross-legged), calming our minds, not sitting with a book and actively scribbling in its pages. But journaling allows us to purge ourselves of stressful thoughts and emotions weighing us down, thereby calming our nervous system and proving to be a useful tool for creating inner peace.

Ironically, journaling often causes people stress at first, because they don't know what to write or they're afraid they might do it wrong. But, I'm here to tell you, there is no right or wrong way to journal. You can write one word, or you can fill ten pages. You can draw pictures to express yourself, or you can give a play-by-play account of your day. On some of the worst days caring for my mom, I would write nothing but "Fuck. Fuck. Fuck. Fuck. Fuck. Fuck. Fuuuuuck!" across the page. Because some days were just those kinds of days.

The beauty of journaling is that it's entirely up to you what you write, but I will offer this: the best way to reap the benefits of stress reduction is to write about the things that are stressing you out. Are you angry because your sibling isn't helping with the caregiving duties? Are you about to scream because your loved one keeps asking you the same question over and over? Do you feel guilty because you yelled at your loved one because they keep asking you the same question? Do you feel that no one acknowledges or appreciates all the sacrifices you are making? Whatever it is, write it down. Don't edit yourself, just go for it. Don't worry if it feels like you're being a Debby Downer and complaining too much. That's what this is for, your journal doesn't mind, it isn't going to judge you. The whole point of journaling is to get it all out so that you aren't walking around carrying all of this junk inside, or worse, dumping it all over the people around you.

Once it's down on paper, you can look at it and digest it differently. Maybe come up with a plan of attack, maybe decide it isn't that bad after all, or maybe acknowledge just how bad it is and realize what a badass you are for being able to hold it all together. When it's outside of you, you have space from what you're experiencing. This space is called "cognitive defusion" and it's what allows you to look at your emotions rather than looking at the world *through* your emotions. It's similar to mindfulness, where you're noticing what your senses are experiencing by taking your emotions out of the equation, except with cognitive defusion, you aren't using your five senses as much as you're using your noggin and your deductive reasoning.

Let's say there are days when you just don't have anything to complain about—great! Write about the dream vacation you'd like to take to reward yourself for all your hard work. Or start writing about what you're grateful for, because there is a profound power in gratitude. Remember that quantum physics theory—what you focus on you create more of? Well, it works with gratitude, too. So, why wouldn't you want more of what you're grateful for?

Pity Parties

I, for one, am a big fan of pity parties. I think there are times in our lives, especially when you're a caregiver, that it's absolutely normal to feel sorry for yourself. Unless being a caregiver is your chosen profession, chances are it wasn't on your bucket list. Your life just got sidelined, and it's a big responsibility—mentally, physically, and financially, and even if you're happy to do it, it's a lot to add to your plate.

We have been taught that feeling sorry for ourselves is a self-indulgent, destructive activity that we shouldn't engage in. And while I don't believe we should marinate in self-pity for long, I do believe that having a moment where you acknowledge how much a situation you are in might suck is very important. Especially when you're a caregiver. Pretending that the situation isn't awful won't help make that situation better. Nor will dismissing your feelings about it. So, why shouldn't you feel sorry for yourself from time to time? I emphatically say, go ahead!

Wallow in it, scream into a pillow, go put on that movie that always makes you bawl and cry your eyes out. Do whatever it is you need to do to process whatever it is that you need to process. It's not doing you or anybody else any good to keep all of that bottled up inside. But then, like any good partygoer, you need to know when it's time to leave.

While I am totally pro-pity party, you need to remember it's a party, not a staycation. It's a limited amount of time you are giving yourself to acknowledge your feelings of overwhelm, frustration, and sadness (for yourself and your loved one), but you are not, and I repeat, you are not moving into that sad space full-time. You need to have your party, then clean up and move on.

How are you supposed to do that? My number one antidote for feeling sorry for myself is to start listing everything I'm grateful for. Either out loud or on paper. Even if you're only grateful for your voice, or the pen in your hand, there is always something to be grateful for. As harsh as this sounds, no matter how bad you think you have it, I guarantee there is someone, somewhere, who would be grateful to have your life.

Self-Care Last Thoughts

Self-care is not selfish. In fact, it's an essential part of being able to take care of others.

We cannot give, help, or provide for anyone else if we're exhausted and falling apart. So, it's imperative that as a caregiver you take some time every day to take care of yourself.

I started with my daily Zen-in-Ten rituals mainly because the idea of taking care of myself for anything longer than ten minutes seemed too frivolous and daunting. But what I didn't know at the time was that just ten minutes of meditation or mindfulness daily, over a period of time, can actually change your brain activity. It can also lower your heart rate, your blood pressure, your adrenaline levels, and your cortisol levels. Thus altering the stress response in your body and possibly diminishing feelings of anxiety.

If you already have a self-care ritual, fantastic! I hope I've given you a couple of ideas to add to that, or if you're a beginner, a place to begin so you can be inspired to give it shot. Really, what do you have to lose except maybe ten minutes and potentially a boat load of cortisol and anxiety?

Your Self-Care Checklist

☐ **Boundaries**—Get them, set them, enforce them! Having established boundaries is a way we show both ourselves and others that we respect our time, our energy, and our emotional well-being. They help define what we are willing and/or capable of doing as a caregiver.

☐ **Mindfulness**—The idea is to be fully aware of your body, your surroundings, and your thoughts in a nonjudgmental way. It's engaging all your senses and fully taking stock of the moment and checking in with reality.

☐ **Meditation**—This is a practice you do to go inward and connect with yourself with the intention of expanding your consciousness and calming your mind.

☐ **Journaling**—Writing allows you to release all of your thoughts and emotions in a safe, nonjudgmental way. The long-term benefits can help reduce stress, improve immune function, lower blood pressure, improve liver function, and improve overall psychological well-being.

☐ **Pity Parties**—I believe a good ol' fashioned Pity Party can be just what the doctor ordered some days. Just don't get too comfortable. No one likes a party goer that overstays their welcome.

Final Thoughts & Wishes

My intention in sharing what I learned during my caregiving escapades is that this book inspires, empowers, and helps you thrive as a caregiver. Knowledge is power, and power is something we very often feel we are lacking when we're caring for a sick or aging loved one. The twists and turns the journey takes can make us feel confused and overwhelmed at times, so my hope is that this book helps prepare you for those moments by offering you information, clarity, and peace of mind when you feel most lost.

That said, it has been my experience that there are some people who will refuse to follow the kind of sound, practical advice I offer in this book. It could be because they believe that by preparing for the worst, they are somehow evoking it. Or maybe they're just the type of person that needs to experience something first before they believe it can happen to them. Regardless, if you're sharing caregiving duties with someone like this, it can be very frustrating and cause a lot of additional stress at a time when tensions are already running high. My suggestion is that you take on the tasks that require immediate attention—like getting the necessary legal documents signed—so at least you've got those bases covered in the case of an emergency.

If it's your loved one that you're caring for who is refusing to cooperate, then perhaps you can explain to them that you're just trying to get all of the unpleasantries out of the way so that the rest of the time you spend together can be enjoyable, quality time.

Because let's face it, nothing we've discussed in this book is fun or easy for anyone involved. Caregiving is an emotionally exhausting endeavor at best, and a heartbreaking ordeal at worst. But, I believe, if you do it right, you can create some calm in the midst of the chaos, and that, my friend, is everything.

So be gentle with yourself, patient with your loved ones, and please, whatever you do, don't compare your journey to anyone else's.

You got this!

Resources for Caregivers

Helpful websites mentioned in this book:

www.AARP.org
AARP is a great resource for most questions you may have about caring for an aging loved one. They also have a Scams and Fraud page so that you can keep on top of Elder Fraud Scams.

www.aginginplace.org
Aging In Place is a wonderful organization for people who want to, well…age in place. Think of it as the Consumer Reports for older adults and caregivers.

www.alz.org
The Alzheimer's Association website has everything from soup to nuts that you may want, and not want, to know about Alzheimer's.

www.fbi.gov
The FBI also has a Scams and Safety page that can help you identify current scams and inform you on how to protect your loved one from becoming a victim to a scam. Search for Elder Fraud.

www.LongTermCare.gov

This website is a good resource for anyone interested in learning more about what Long-Term Care options they may have.

As luck would have it, it happens to be a part of The Administration for Community Living website (www.acl.gov), whose mission is to help individuals, regardless of age or disability, live healthy, independent lives. So it's a twofer for those looking for long-term care information.

www.Medicaid.gov

This government website has all the information you need about your state's Medicaid coverage. Buyer beware, it can be a bit frustrating to navigate, so be patient and don't start your search if you're already stressed out or in a rush. Just sayin'.

www.Medicare.gov

If you're living in the United States and are over the age of sixty-five, then you are most likely familiar with this website. Still, I just wanted to include it in case, after reading this book, you were interested in learning more about specific insurance options—like Medigap, for instance.

Not mentioned in this book, but a good resource for caregivers who need a much needed break:

www.archrespite.org

The ARCH National Respite Network and Resource Center is an advocacy organization dedicated to helping family caregivers find respite programs in their communities.

From Zero to Zen
Master Checklist

I'm a big fan of the saying "get your ducks in a row"—as you may have gathered by my use of the term multiple times in this book. In my opinion, not only is it a nicer way of saying, "Get your shit together," it also conjures up images of happy little duck families peacefully swimming along in a single file. And who doesn't love that?

The thing about ducks though, is that as calm and peaceful as they may seem floating about, their little webbed feet are paddling a mile a minute below the surface. *From Zero to Zen* is about giving you the information and tools you need as a caregiver to be prepared so that you can remain calm, but you're still going to be paddling like hell behind the scenes to make sure everything is taken care of so you can stay afloat.

So, in the name of tools, paddling, and maintaining a Zen-like calm, I've put together a Master Checklist that includes all the information you will need, and even some information you may not need but should still probably have. Just. In. Case.

I've also made an expanded version of this list available for free on my website. Go to www.alexandrafree.com and download your free PDF version of *The Caregiver's Master Checklist* and start getting all those duckies together!

The Caregiver's Master Checklist

PERSONAL HISTORY

Name: ____

Birth Name: ____

Date of Birth:________________Place of Birth:________________

Adopted: YES______NO______Adoption Date: ________________

Additional Adoption Information:________________________

Current Address: ____________________________________

How Many Years at Current Residence: ________________

Phone Number(s):____________________________________

Email Address:______________________________________

Social Security Number:______________________________

Driver License Number:________Expiration:________State Issued:______

Passport Number:________Expiration:________Country Issued:________

MILITARY SERVICE

Veteran: YES______NO______

Branch of Military:__________________________________

Rank:__________________Serial Number: ________________

Type of Discharge: __________________________________

Medals of Distinction:_______________________________

Additional Information:______________________________

____

____

____

EDUCATIONAL BACKGROUND

Elementary School:_______________________________________

Town & State:____

Junior High School:______________________________________

Town & State:____

Highschool:____

Town & State:____

College(s):____

Town & State:____

Major/Degree:____

MARITAL STATUS

Married ☐ Divorced ☐ Widowed ☐ Single ☐

Name of Spouse:____

Phone Number(s):_______________________________________

Email Address:____

Spouse's Birthday:________________Place of Birth:___________

Wedding date:________________Wedding Location:___________

Date of Spouse's Death: _________________________________

Where is Spouse Buried/Interred: _________________________

Address:____

Additional Spouse Information: ___________________________

____

____

____

____

CHILDREN

How Many Children:____

Child's Name:____

Child's Birthday:_____________________________Place of Birth:______________

Child's Current Address:____

Phone Number(s):____

Email Address:____

Where they went to school:____

Occupation:____

Current Employer:____

Is Child Married: YES________NO________

Child's Spouse:____

Spouse's Birthday:____

Wedding date:____

Phone Number(s):____

Email Address:____

GRANDCHILDREN

How Many Grandchildren:____

Grandchild's Name:____

Grandchild's Parents:____

Grandchild's Birthday:____

Address:____

Phone Number(s):____

Email Address:____

Grandchild's Name:____________________________________

Grandchild's Parents:________________________________

Grandchild's Birthday:________________________________

Address:____

Phone Number(s):___________________________________

Email Address:______________________________________

Grandchild's Name:____________________________________

Grandchild's Parents:________________________________

Grandchild's Birthday:________________________________

Address:____

Phone Number(s): ___________________________________

Email Address:______________________________________

LEGAL DOCUMENTS

☐ Durable Power of Attorney (POA): YES______NO______

Type of POA: Financial POA ☐ Medical POA ☐ Both ☐

Is a HIPAA waiver included? YES______NO______

Name of POA(s):____________________________________

Phone Number(s):____________________________________

Email Address:______________________________________

☐ Health Care Proxy: YES______NO______

Is a HIPAA waiver included? YES______NO______

Name of Proxy:_____________________________________

Phone Number(s):____________________________________

Email Address:______________________________________

☐ A Living Will: YES______NO______

Who has a copy? ____

☐ An Advance Healthcare Directive: YES______NO______

Who has a copy?____

☐ A Do Not Resuscitate Order (DNR): YES______NO______

☐ A Do Not Intubate Order (DNI): YES______NO______

☐ A Will: YES______NO______

Name of Executor/Executrix of the Will:___________________________

Phone Number(s):____

Email Address:____

☐ A Living Trust: YES______NO______

Name of Trustee:____

Phone Number(s):____

Email Address:____

☐ Marriage License: YES______NO______

Where is it?____

☐ Divorce Papers: YES______NO______

Where are they?____

Additional Information: ____

____

____

____

NAMES & CONTACT INFORMATION FOR ALL ATTORNEYS

Name of Attorney:____

Law Firm:____

Type of Attorney:____

Phone Number(s):____

Email Address:____

Name of Attorney:____

Law Firm:____

Type of Attorney:____

Phone Number(s):____

Email Address:____

MEDICAL INFORMATION

☐ Medications:

Name of Medication & dosage:_____________________________________

What it is for:____

Name of Medication & dosage:_____________________________________

What it is for:____

Name of Medication & dosage:_____________________________________

What it is for:____

Name of Medication & dosage:_____________________________________

What it is for:____

Name of Medication & dosage:_____________________________________

What it is for:____

Name of Medication & dosage:____

What it is for:____

Name of Medication & dosage:____

What it is for:____

☐ **Blood Type:**____

☐ **Allergies:**____

Food Allergies:____

Medication Allergies:____

☐ **Medical Records & Results:** ____

Where are the records kept?____

Test performed: ____

Results & Date: ____

Test performed: ____

Results & Date: ____

Test performed: ____

Results & Date: ____

Test performed: ____

Results & Date: ____

Test performed: ____

Results & Date: ____

Test performed: ____

Results & Date: ____

NAMES & CONTACT INFORMATION FOR ALL PHYSICIANS:

Name of Doctor:_______________________________________

Type of Doctor: _______________________________________

Phone Number(s): _______________________________________

Email Address:: _______________________________________

Name of Doctor:_______________________________________

Type of Doctor: _______________________________________

Phone Number(s): _______________________________________

Email Address:: _______________________________________

Name of Doctor:_______________________________________

Type of Doctor: _______________________________________

Phone Number(s): _______________________________________

Email Address:: _______________________________________

Name of Doctor:_______________________________________

Type of Doctor: _______________________________________

Phone Number(s): _______________________________________

Email Address:: _______________________________________

Additional Information:_______________________________________

____

____

____

____

____

HEALTH INSURANCE INFORMATION

Medicare: Medicare Number:____

Which Plan(s): Part A ☐ Part B ☐ Part C (Medicare Advantage) ☐
          Part D ☐

☐ Medicare Advantage Insurance Provider:: _____________________

Phone Number(s): _______________________________________

Email Address:: ____

☐ Gap Insurance: YES______NO______Policy Number: _______________

Gap Insurance Provider:__________________________________

Phone Number(s): ____

Email Address:: ____

☐ Long-Term Care Insurance: YES______NO______
Policy Number:____

LTCI Insurance Provider:__________________________________

Phone Number(s):____

Email Address: ____

☐ Medicaid Insurance: YES_____NO_____Medicaid Number: ___________

Medicaid Caseworker:____________________________________

Phone Number(s):____

Email Address:____

Additional Information:___________________________________

____

____

____

____

OTHER INSURANCE INFORMATION

☐ Auto Insurance: YES______NO______Policy Number:__________________

Insurance Provider:____

Phone Number(s):________________Email Address: __________________

☐ Homeowner's Insurance: YES____NO______Policy Number:____________

Insurance Provider:____

Phone Number(s):____

Email Address:____

☐ Renter's Insurance: YES______NO______Policy Number:______________

Insurance Provider:____

Phone Number(s):____

Email Address:____

☐ Life Insurance: YES______NO______Policy Number:__________________

Is there a cash value? YES______NO______Cash Value: ________________

Insurance Provider: ____

Phone Number(s):____

Email Address:____

Additional Information:____

____

____

____

____

____

____

FINANCIAL INFORMATION

☐ **Assets:**

Property (primary residence):_______________________________________

Property Value (approx.): ____

Amount Owed on Mortgage:____

Other Properties: Vacation ☐ Rental ☐ Business ☐ Timeshare ☐
Other ☐

Property Value (approx.):____

Amount Owed on Mortgage:____

Property Value (approx.):____

Amount Owed on Mortgage: ____

☐ **Personal Property:**____

Automobile(s): Own ☐ Lease ☐

Make, Model, Year & Approximate Value:______________________________

____

Antiques: Item(s) & Approximate Value:_______________________________

____

Art, Jewelry & Collectibles: Item(s) & Approximate Value: _______________

____

Miscellaneous: Item(s) & Approximate Value:__________________________

____

☐ **Source(s) of Income: Total Monthly Amount:**____________________

Salary:_______________Pensions:_______________401K:_____________

IRA:_______________Trusts:_______________Investments:_____________

Settlements: ____

Social Security:_______________Other:______________________________

BANKING ACCOUNTS

☐ Savings Account Number:____

Bank & Branch: ____

Online Banking Login Username:____

Password:____

☐ Checking Account Number:____

Bank & Branch:____

Online Banking Login Username:____

Password:____

☐ Money Market Account Number:____

Bank & Branch:____

Online Banking Login Username:____

Password:____

☐ Certificate of Deposit (CD) Account Number:____________________________

Bank & Branch:____

Online Banking Login Username:____

Password:____

☐ Safety Deposit Box: YES______NO______Is there a co-owner?

YES______NO______

Do you have the documents to access the Safety Deposit Box?

YES______NO______

Bank & Branch:____

Where is the key?____

Contents:____

____

Acknowledgments

Caregiving takes a village, and I would not have been able to care for my parents without the love, support and occasional cocktails provided by mine. My Village (in no particular order):

The Sponheimer Clan:

Matt, David and John: You have been there for me from the moment I took my first breath (well, at least Matt and David were, John you came along a little later). You've made being an only child feel like a group sport and I could write books about how much each of you means to me. But I won't. Not yet.

Yasmin, Nicole and Kelley: You are the sisters I never had and, although your taste in men is questionable, I'm forever grateful you married my cousins and came into my life.

Uncle Bob and Anne: You were there for me every step of the way be it with advice, support or a much needed night out on the town. There are no words to express my gratitude for all you have done for me.

Andrea: Thank you for being a second mother to me right from the very start and for always telling me I earned "every star in my crown" while caring for Mom—it truly meant the world to me.

Ella, Brianna, Alia, Karim, Max, Sam, Jack, and Sean: Thank you for making me an aunt and for giving me a reason to smile at a time when I often had little to smile about.

The rest of my tribe:

Elsie and Kenneth X. Free: Thank you for keeping the Free fires burning. Your love, support and oranges mean everything.

Eileen DePaoli: Thank you for always having my back and for making sure I had Gluten Free options even before it was easy.

Claire Buehler, Wendy Jennings and Laurie Heber: Thank you for making me feel like family even before we were. You are the best in-laws a girl could ask for.

Anne Weber: The day I walked into your open house was a very good day indeed. Thank you for becoming my big sister, for sharing your family and for always knowing when I needed hot chocolate therapy.

Miranda Barrett, Stephanie Jourdan and Tarra: I would not have been able to navigate my journey without your guidance, support, insight, love and the magical woo-woo you do.

Alex Weed, Amy Capuano, Angie Sutthoff, Hope Boyd, Janice Sampson, Kerry Fitzmaurice, Kim Schwarzkopf and Lisa Hawkins: Thank you for being my extended family, my partners in crime and my shoulders to cry on. There is no way to sum up how much your friendship means to me except to say—it's been a wild ride and I'm forever grateful you're riding it with me.

My work family: Greg Sills, Cheryl Teetzel-Moore, Meachun Clarke, Andrea Regalado, Michelle Robinson, James Casares, Katie Carlin, Amy Johnson, Paul Flattery, Mo Moroney, Dylan Forer, Stephanie Butler, Joette Phillips, Michael Potts, Brett Ostro, Gary Tellalian, Cheryl Parker and Lynn Lendway: Working with you helped bring light and laughter to some of my darkest hours. I loved every show we did together, even the ones we hated at the time and swore we'd never do again.

My From Zero to Zen family:

Staci Frenes: My editor extraordinaire, you helped make this dream a reality and found the words when I couldn't.

Christy Day: Your design skills are second to none—except possibly your patience.

To everyone who inspired this book, championed the idea when it was just a pipe dream, and then happily grabbed their pompoms when I needed cheering on—I am eternally grateful.

And finally:

Lola: My Baby Girl. You were my light in the storm, my reason for getting out of bed and the cutest, sassiest, most wonderful antidote for everything life was throwing at me—thank you for picking me.

Dave: The earth moved the day we met, and it's never stopped shaking. Thank you for giving me the time and space to make this dream a reality and for being the best papa Lola could ask for. I love and appreciate you. Go Giants!

About the Author

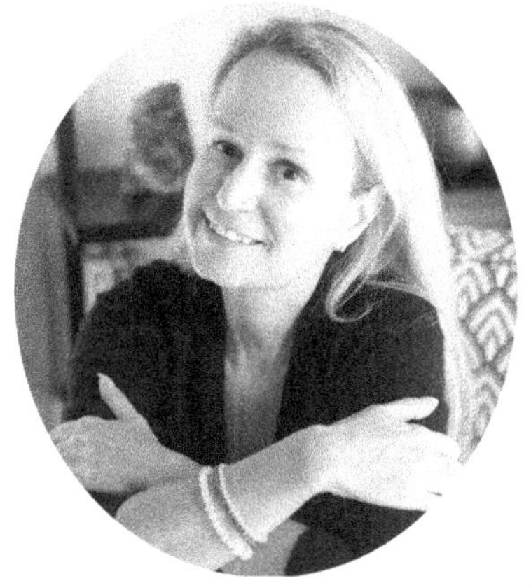

Alexandra Free spent twenty years as a talent executive and stage manager in the demanding field of live television, working with A-list celebrities, producers, publicists, and network executives. But her world turned upside down the day she got a call that her father was in the hospital, and then again when she discovered her mother had Alzheimer's. Over the following decade, she immersed herself in the world of caregiving, learning everything she could to successfully advocate for her parents while also learning—the hard way—the importance self-care plays in the physical and mental well-being of a caregiver.

www.AlexandraFree.com
Instagram: @alexandracfree
Pinterest: @alexandracfree
Facebook: facebook.com/alexandracfree